Unleash The Machine

ISBN: 1-4196-3365-1

To order additional copies, please contact us.
BookSurge, LLC
www.booksurge.com
1-866-308-6235
orders@booksurge.com

Unleash The Machine

A Marine's Guide to Elite Fitness

Bobby L. Clark

2006

Unleash The Machine

TABLE OF CONTENTS

ACKNOWLEDGEMENTS

Throughout my life I have been privileged to work with and for some extremely influential people. Some are family members and friends, some have been coworkers and fellow Marines, and one was my high school wrestling coach. Thanks to these people and to the events that impacted me to the effect of great inspiration, I am the man I am today. So to all of you who taught me to lead by example, to accept failure as a lesson—not a loss, to be passionate towards all of your goals, and last but not least, to be humble in your successes, I thank you.

This Book Is Dedicated To All Those Whom I Have Had The Privilege Of Serving With. . ."Stay Motivated!"

INTRODUCTION

Since you are reading this book, it is goes without saying that you are ready for a change. You should know immediately that this book isn't a "Get Big Quick Plan" or a "Secret Formula" to achieving any level of fitness. It is simply the purest form of natural strength and endurance training you will find.

Since you are still reading, you are ready to experience a life-altering lesson in developing your body and mind into a focused, performance-driven "MACHINE."

First, let me explain the training development with these lessons. Most of the exercises and workouts are based on body-weight manipulation and muscular concentration in order to develop and create the desired affects: strength, muscular development, and endurance. You will be learning basic exercises, which will act as the foundation for your workouts, and you will also learn advanced exercises, which can be conducted once you have developed your level of fitness.

Secondly, let's talk about the advantages of this type of training. As you begin training, regardless of what level of fitness you are in, you will immediately be surprised at the difficulty of some of the exercises. This is the case especially if you are a weight lifter and use to moving much more weight in iron than that of your own body. As you continue your training, you will soon feel the difference in not only your appearance, but in every aspect of yourself. You will notice feeling stronger, more energetic, and better about yourself. The reason for these changes is a result of accomplishing all three aspects of a good physical training plan: muscular strength, muscular endurance, and flexibility. Also—unlike weight lifting—you are developing your muscles to move your body around objects, rather than objects around your body. What does that mean? It means you're you simply are strengthening your core muscles. These are the smaller less noticeable muscles that act as joint stabilizers, therefore enabling your body to build from the inside out. "Hold on there weight lifter! I have nothing against lifting weights; this is simply an alternate way of muscular development." For those of you who still perfer to utilize weight training, this is just an additional tool for your toolbox to give you the advantage over the other guy or girl.

Finally, I need to clarify that the exercises and workouts I have written into this book are designed to develop an extreme level of fitness—both strength and endurance. So consider yourself warned. For those of you who have the desire and the drive to achieve your goal, you will find my guidance to be an asset to training regimen.

"From this point on the gloves are off, so warm-up, stretch out, and *GET SOME!*"

CHAPTER I

SHOULDERS

"If working out were easy, everybody would be in shape"

HANDSTAND PUSH-UPS:

There are three basic variations of handstand push-ups: Back to wall, Face to wall, and "1-3-5" count

NOTE: The handstand push-up is one of the most intense body-weight exercises you will ever experience. For a beginner, you should be proud if you can accomplish just five reps. For someone who is more advanced, fifteen to twenty repetitions should be your goal.

BACK TO WALL: The back to wall handstand push-up exercise is awesome for packing on some density to your deltoids and "traps"(trapezoids).

STEPS:

1) You want to start by facing the wall in a squatting position. Place the palms of your hands down about six to ten inches from the wall, slightly greater than shoulder width apart.
2) Next put the top of your head between your hands and kick up into a headstand. Let your feet catch you against the wall.
3) Now press your body up until your arms are fully extended and supporting your body weight. This is the starting position for the exercise.
4) From this position slowly lower your body down until your nose touches the ground. Do not let your body weight rest on your head and continue to support yourself with your hands and shoulders. This is your half rep.
5) Now with controlled exhalation, press your body straight up, supporting your body weight on the heels and fingertips of you hands until your arms are once again fully extended. You have just completed one rep.

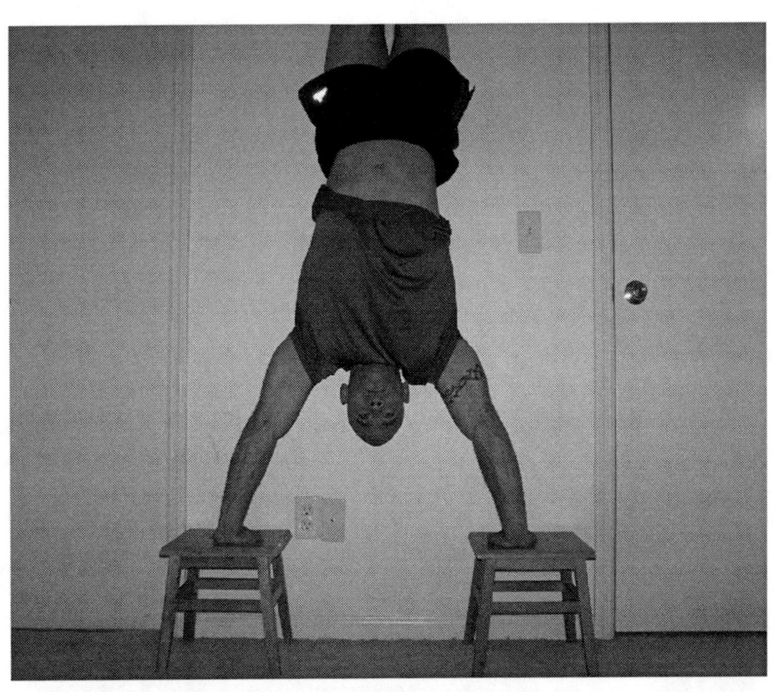

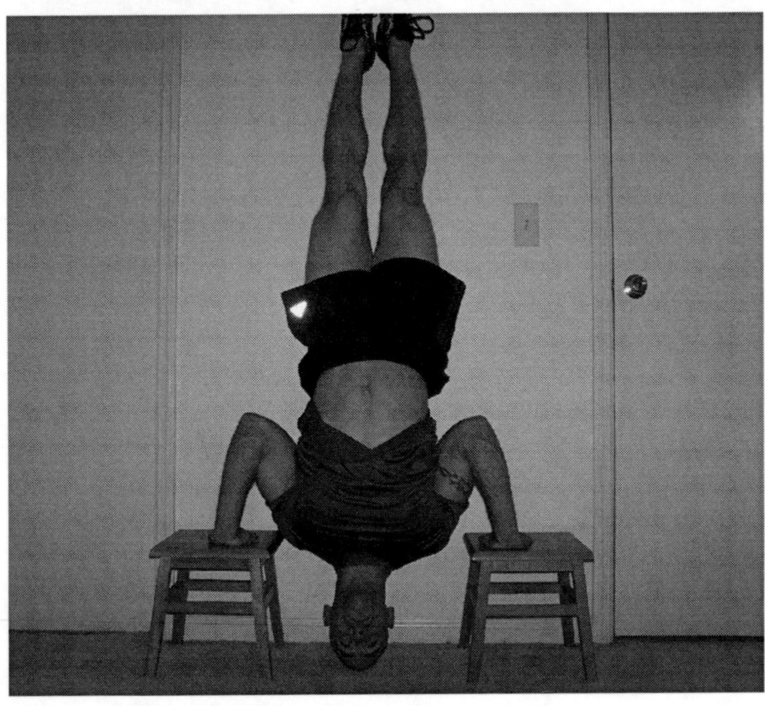

FACE TO WALL: These develop a powerful, and not to mention, muscular shape to the front of your deltoids and the top of your chest.

STEPS:

1) Start by standing with your back to the wall. Squat down and place your hands on the ground palms down, slightly wider than shoulder width apart.
2) Next walk your feet up the wall until your body is completely straight.
3) Then walk your hands in towards the wall until they are about six inches away. This is your starting position.
4) Rep one is done by slowly lowering your body, allowing the top of your feet to slide down with your body. Control your descend all the way down until your nose touches the ground.
5) Now explode up with controlled exhalation back to the starting position. Allow your feet to naturally slide back up the wall. YOU MUST KEEP YOUR BODY STRAIGHT! Good job, rep one is complete. Now keep pounding them out.

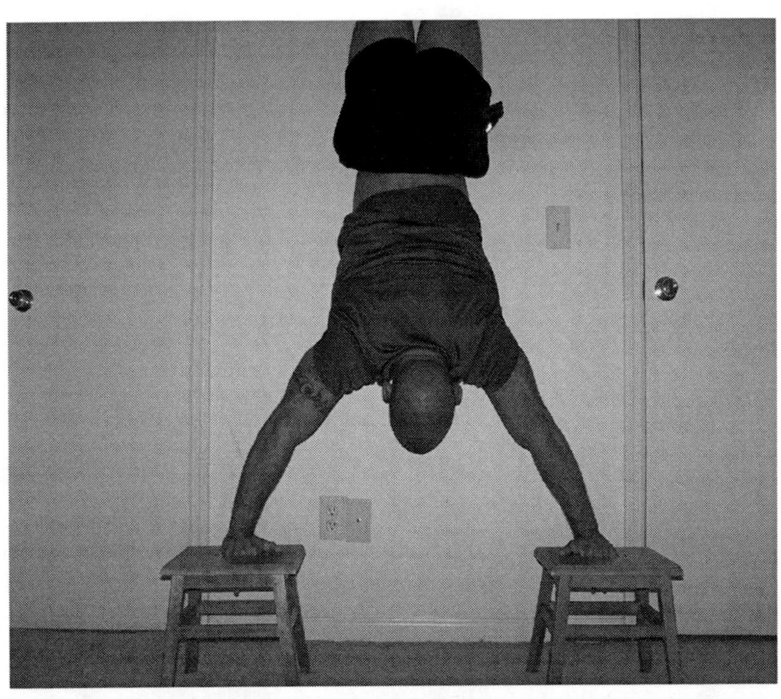

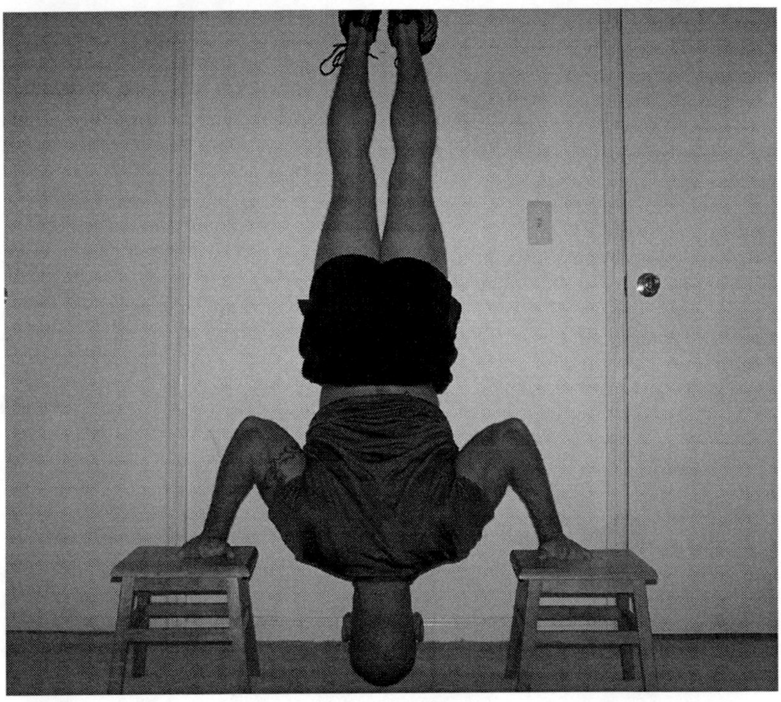

"5-3-1" HANDSTAND PUSH-UPS: These can be done with either version of the handstand push-up. The developmental principal behind this technique is complete controlled isolation.

STEPS:

1) Begin in either starting position. Next lower yourself down to the half position at a speed of a five-second count. Your nose should be as close to the ground as it can be without actually touching.
2) Now hold this position for three seconds. Once you reach three seconds, explode up with a controlled exhalation for a count of one second.
3) You should now be back in the starting position. Remember don't cheat the count.

NOTE: Controlled exhalation is extremely important when conducting these exercises. Due to the position of the body, extreme pressure is exerted in your head and face. *So if you feel your eyeballs about to pop, STOP!*

A LITTLE MORE: The exercises we have just completed are great, but they can be improved by utilizing elevation (as seen in the above pictures). Simply take two chairs, blocks, or stools and place them against the wall. From here, place your hands on the chairs instead of the floor. Conduct the handstand push-up from the chair, stool, or block, and the intensity is multiplied. A couple key points: Go slow, Go deep, and Breathe!!! You'll notice that you can go much farther down (Go Deep!), and your capability will be greatly reduced at first. That is until you build your strength to handle this much resistance. Go slow and train hard.

HINDU PUSH-UPS: Not to be confused with dive-bomber push-ups. These bad boys get the blood flowing, and the shoulders burning. There are two different positions for this exercise. One position is good for beginners, and the second position is for the real "MACHINES" out there.

POSITION ONE:

STEPS:

1) Start with your feet spread out MUCH WIDER than your shoulders.
2) Next place your hands flat on the ground in front of you about shoulder width apart. Your body should make an upside down V.

NOTE: The closer your feet are to your hands, the more difficult the exercise will be.

3) Now, simply look between your legs by pushing until your arms and shoulders are completely straight. This is your starting position.
4) In an arcing motion, bend your arms allowing your nose, followed by your chest, then your hips to graze the ground until you are looking at the sky with your arms once again straight. Your hips should be hovering above the ground just behind your hands. This is half a rep
5) Now without bending your arms, use your shoulders to push your butt back in the air and back in the starting position. Make sure you look deep between your legs, giving your shoulders a good squeeze. Rep one complete, now rep out as many as you can.

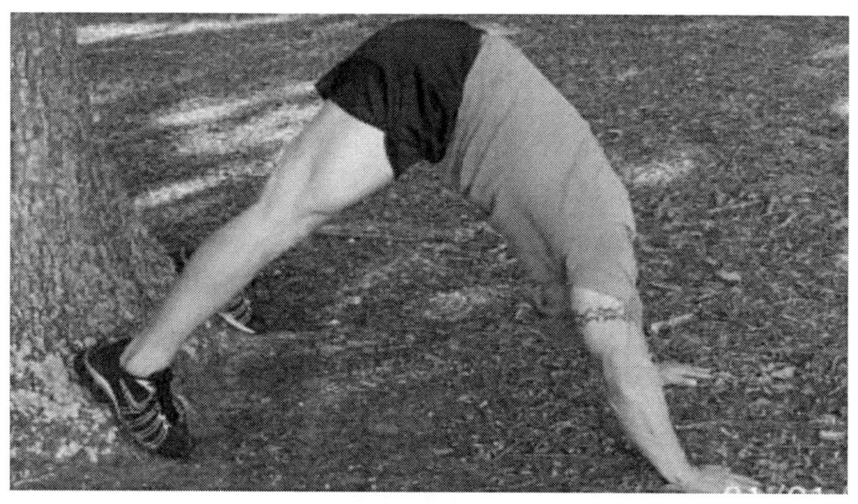

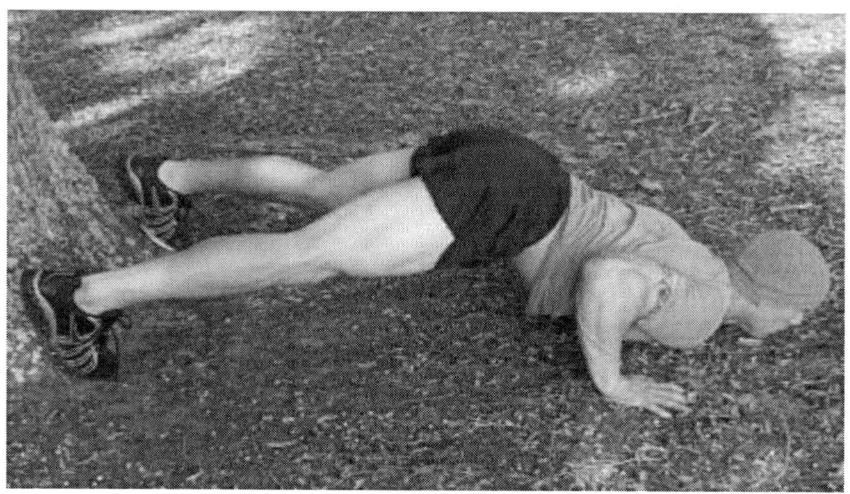

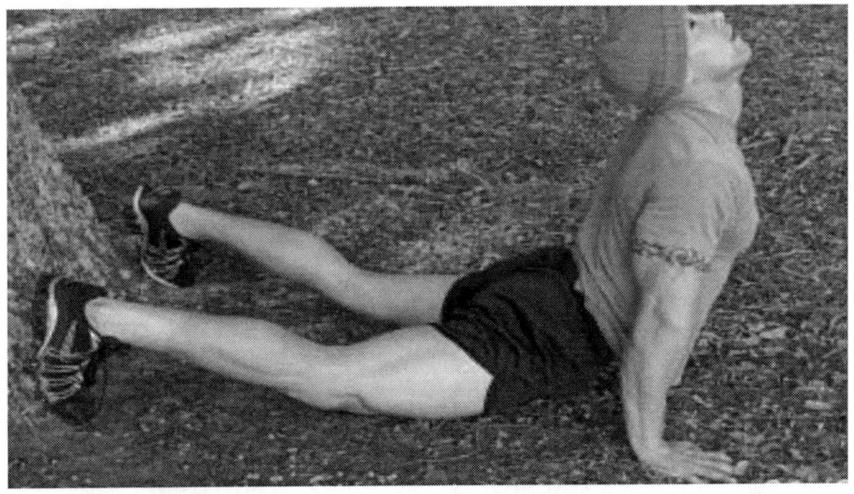

POSTION TWO: Okay now that we know what we're doing, let's see how tough we really are. Find yourself a wall (or a tree as in the picture above) and take the starting position for position one—except place the bottom of you feet flat against the wall. Now the only things touching the ground are your toes and hands. This puts twice the amount of body weight and pressure on your shoulders. The key is not to cheat, so keep that extra weight on your hands. Breath through every rep and you're well on your way to developing strong wide shoulders.

PRESS-UPS: This exercise focuses on the front of the shoulders and part of the upper chest. You will need something (I chose a sandbag) to elevate your hands off the deck.

<u>**STEPS:**</u>

1) Start out with your feet flat against the wall and your hands on the sandbag. You body should look similar to a push-up position accept your butt is high in the air like an inverted V.
2) Now your hands should be some what close and inline with your chest. Your head should be just ahead of the sandbag.
3) Now from here simply lower yourself down until your chest touches the sandbag. Keep your elbows in tight to you body.
4) From here press up, exhaling at the same time and pressing your body back up into the starting position. That's one rep, now pump them out.

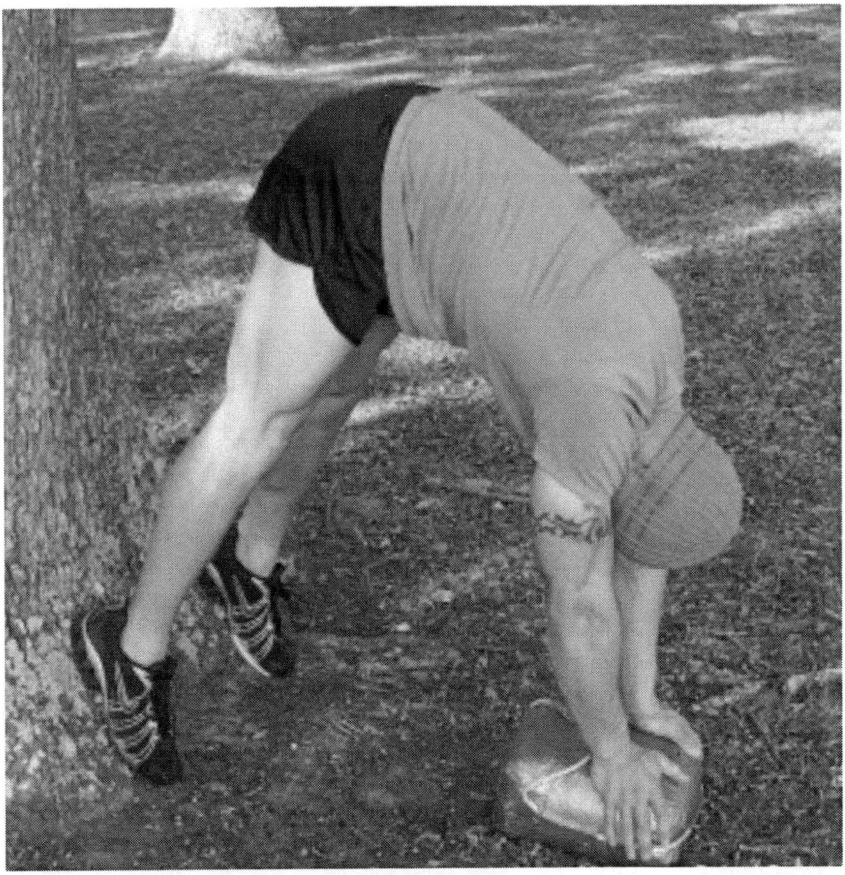

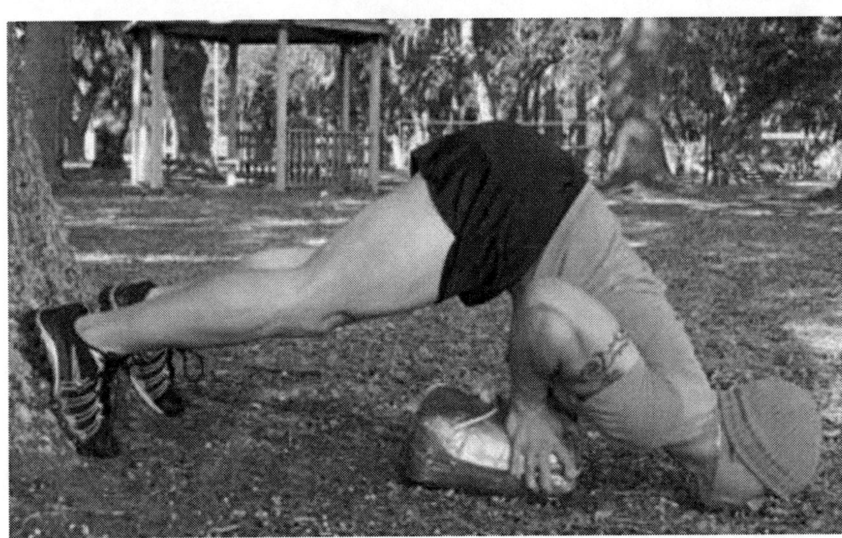

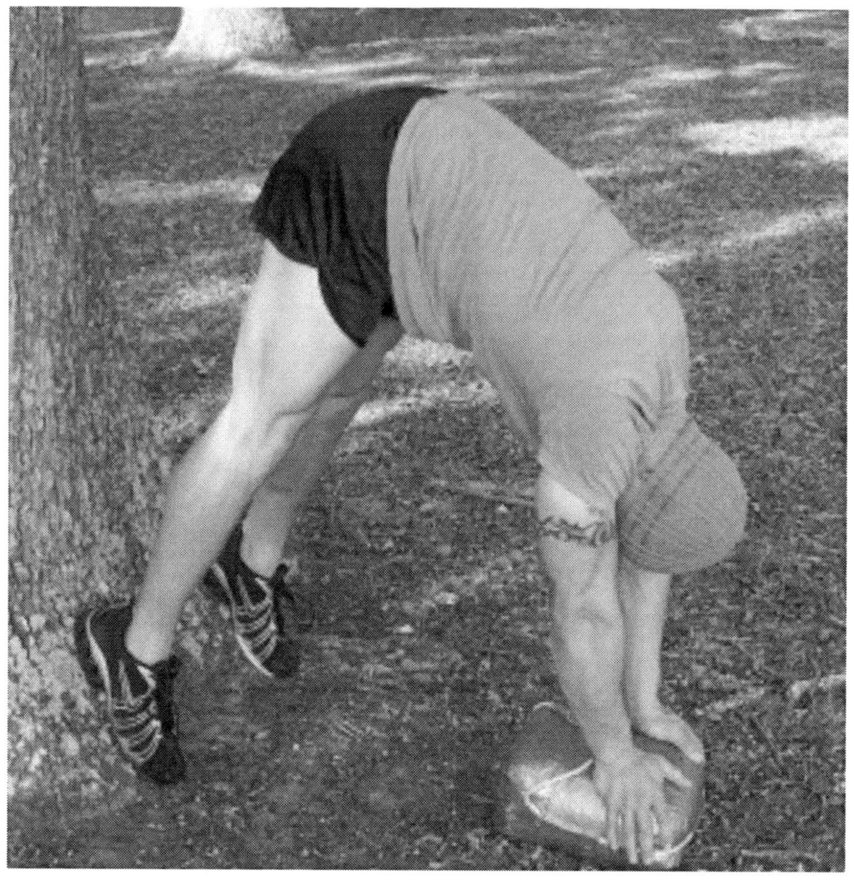

CHAPTER 2

BICEPS

"The results are worth the grueling effort, not to mention the pain."

All right, before we get in to the actual exercise, let's talk about grip. As you've already realized, pull-ups work mainly the lats, forearms, and inner back. Well that's because you are minimizing the stress applied to the biceps by utilizing your thumb in your grip. Now for the next four exercises we do, we are simply going to eliminate the thumb from the grip. So rather than griping the bar with a full grasp, ensuring that your palms are facing you, take your thumbs and place them on the same side of the bar as your fingers. Now let's destroy our "bi's."

ISOLATED PULL-UPS:

STEPS:

1) The starting position of your hands is anywhere from twelve inches to touching, measured from the inside of your grip (depending on your frame and flexibility).
2) Your legs should be slightly extended in front of your body with your elbows fully locked. Now, ensuring that you squeeze your elbows in tight as if you were trying to touch them together, pull your chin to the bar utilizing only your biceps. This is where the control comes into play. You can accomplish this, pausing halfway up for one second, and then completing the movement.
3) Once at the top, pause for a second as you flex your biceps to full peak. That is a half rep. Now simply lower your body down to the starting position, once again concentrating on your biceps.
4) Once your elbows are completely extended, STOP. Your back should not be used through this entire exercise. The KEY to isolating your biceps is accomplished by only going far enough down to extend the arms, not your shoulders and back, while attempting to eliminate the lats from the exercise. Now go until failure and feel the difference.

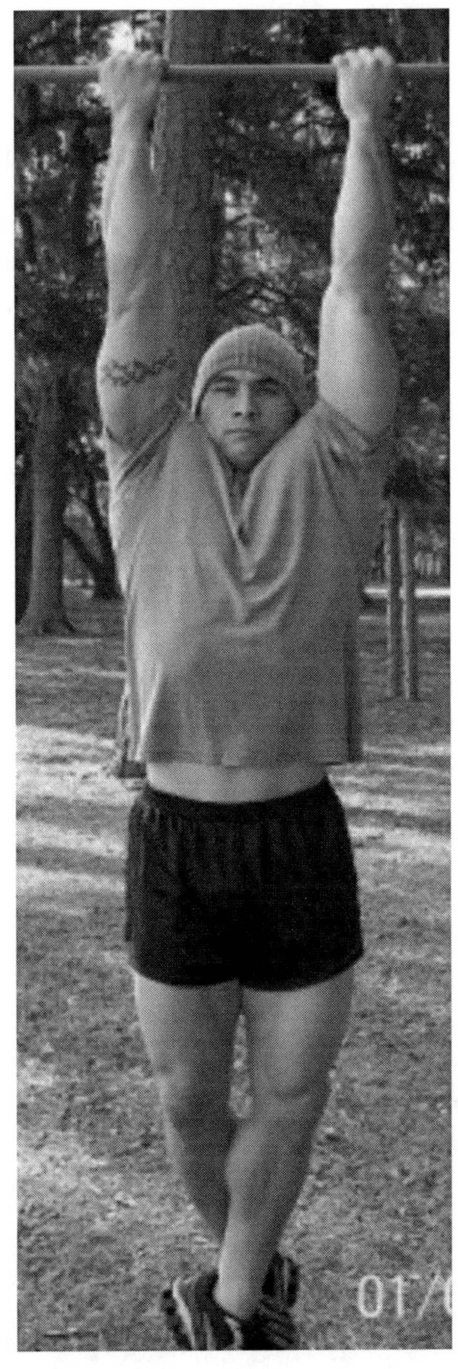

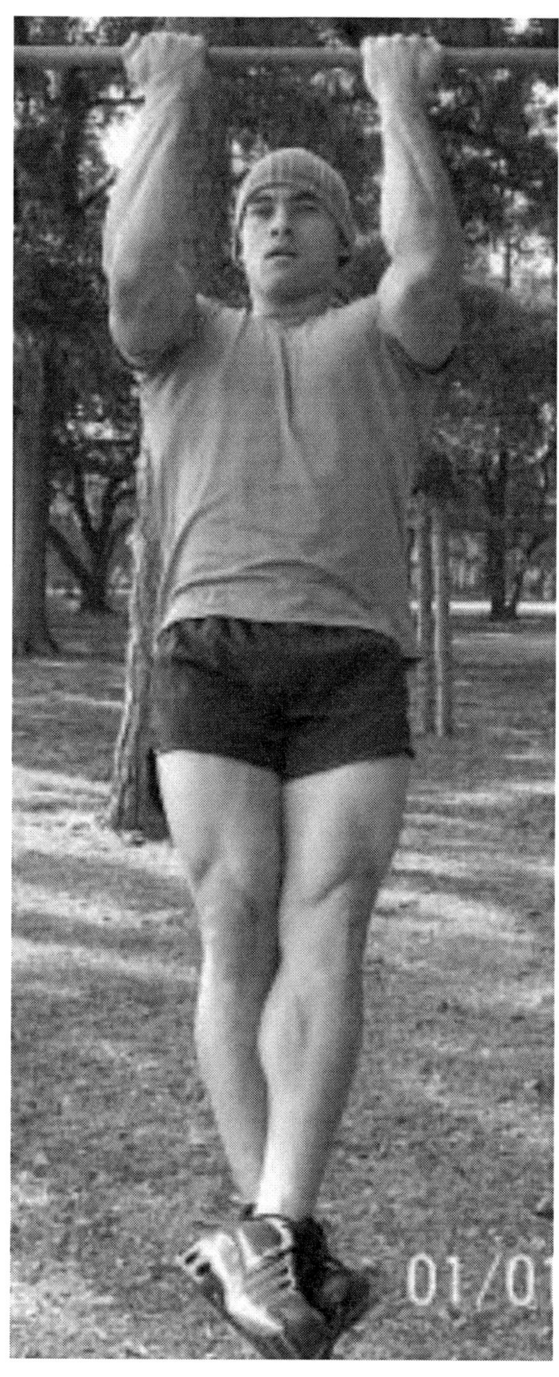

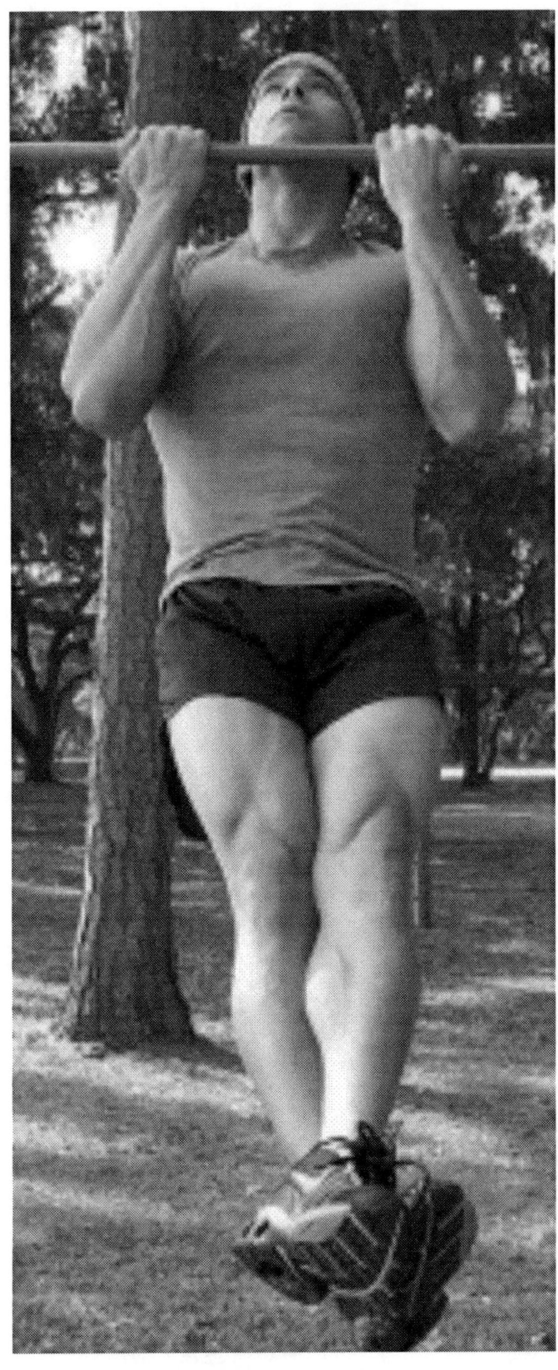

1-3-5 PULL-UPS: This exercises principal is based from the *ISOLATION PULL-UPS.* Utilizing the same starting position, ascent and descent principals, simple apply the count. So the single rep will be as follows.

STEPS:

1) Starting position (arms fully extended). Pull up to the half rep (chin to the bar) at a pace of a one count.
2) Pause and squeeze for a three count.
3) Then descend at a rate of a five count.

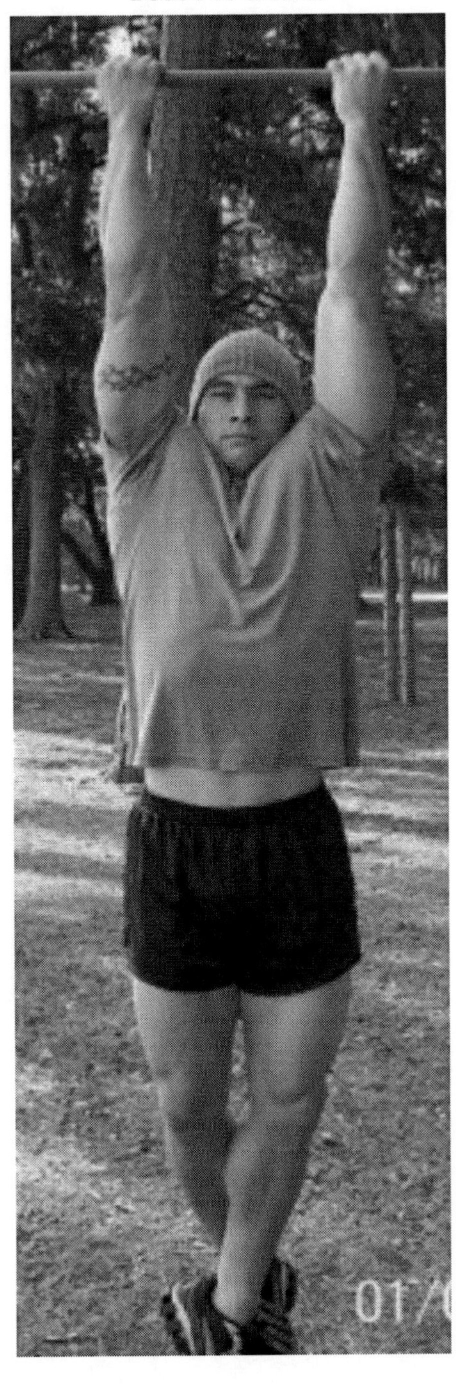
01/

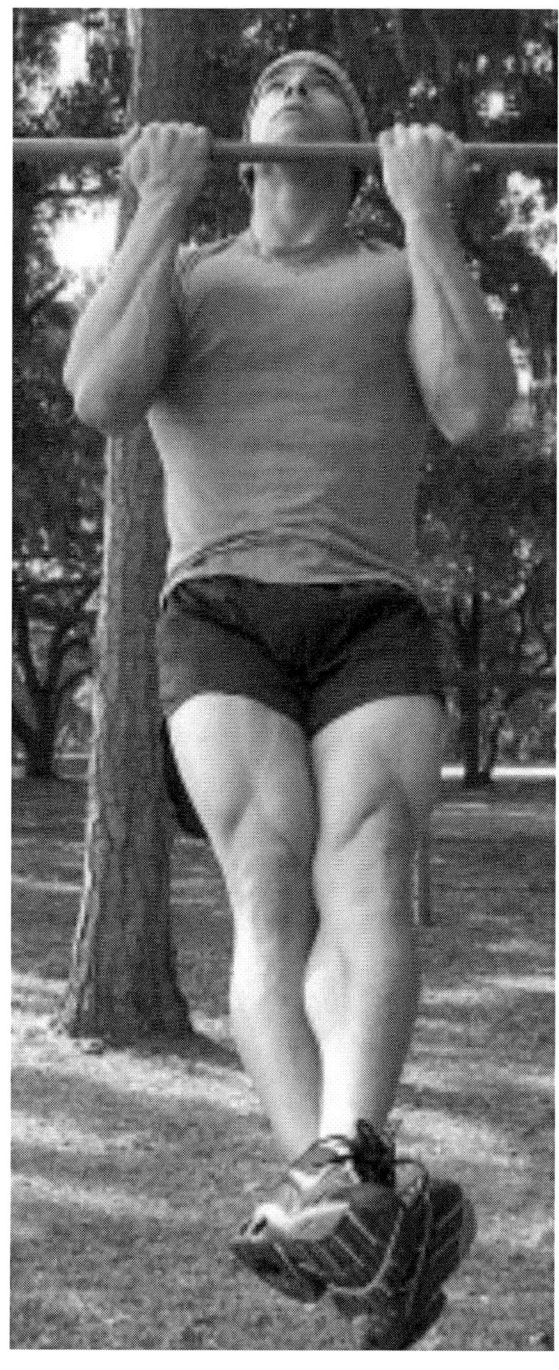

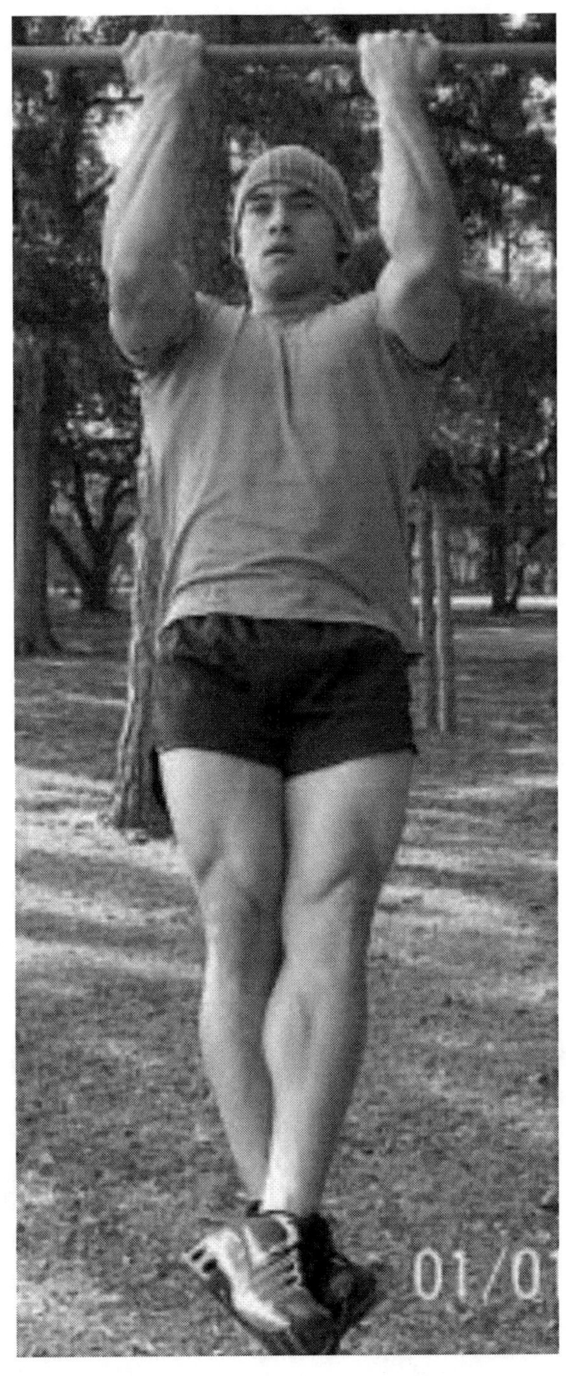

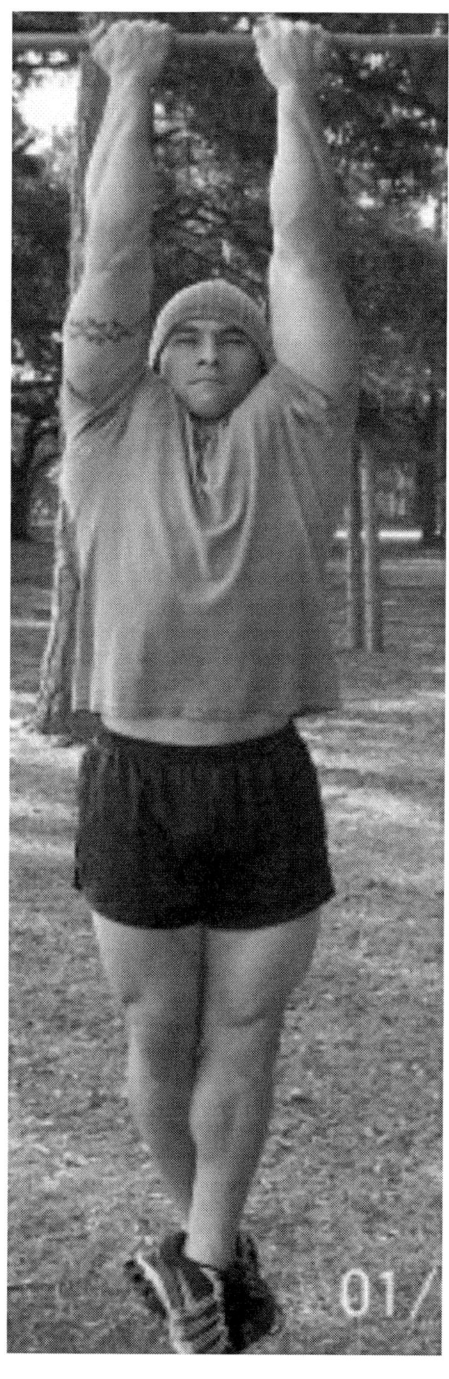
01/

FIFTEENS: This exercise is a great way to start or finish a work out. Whether it it's to get the blood flowing with a great initial pump, or to finish them off by destroying the muscle from every possible angle. Sounds fun doesn't it? Okay, once again all *ISOLATION PULL-UP* principals apply. The key this time is in the motion.

<u>**STEPS:**</u>

1) Go ahead and pull yourself up to half rep (chin to the bar).
2) Now on your descent only go down halfway (arms at ninety degrees), then go back up again. That's rep one. Do a total of five from the top.
3) Now, once you've completed your first five reps, lower yourself back down to the starting position (arms fully extended).
4) From here you are going to pull up, but you stop at the halfway point (ninety degrees). See the pattern yet? Now do a total of five reps at the bottom. Hang in there; now that's ten reps. We still have five more reps.
5) Return to the starting position (arms fully extended). The last five reps are the best. Now all you have to do is complete five more reps of the basic *ISOLATON PULL-UP,* all the way up, and all the way down. Now that's just one set. Talk about a pump!

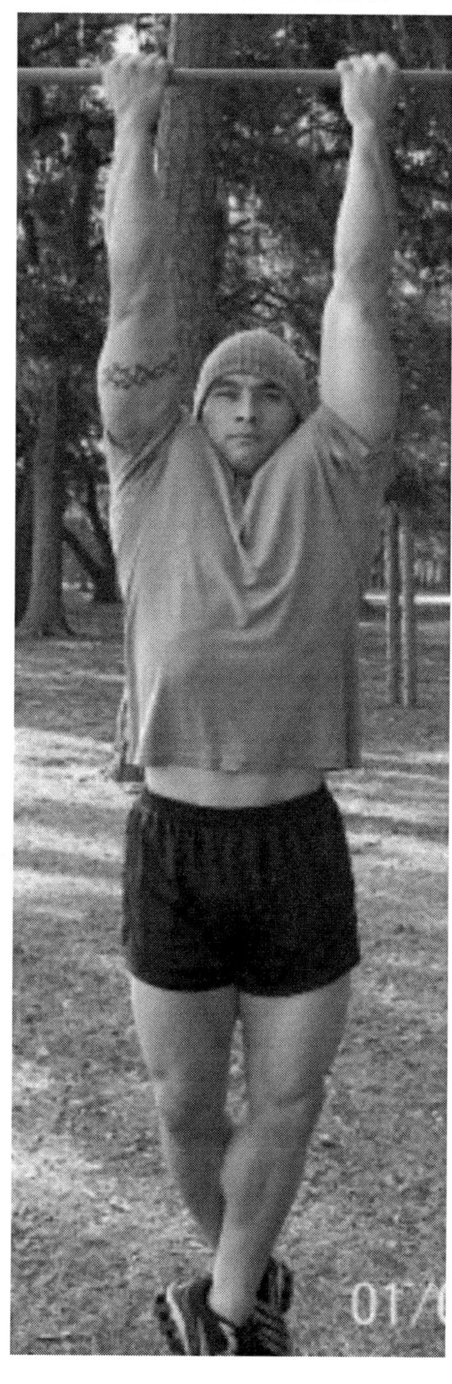

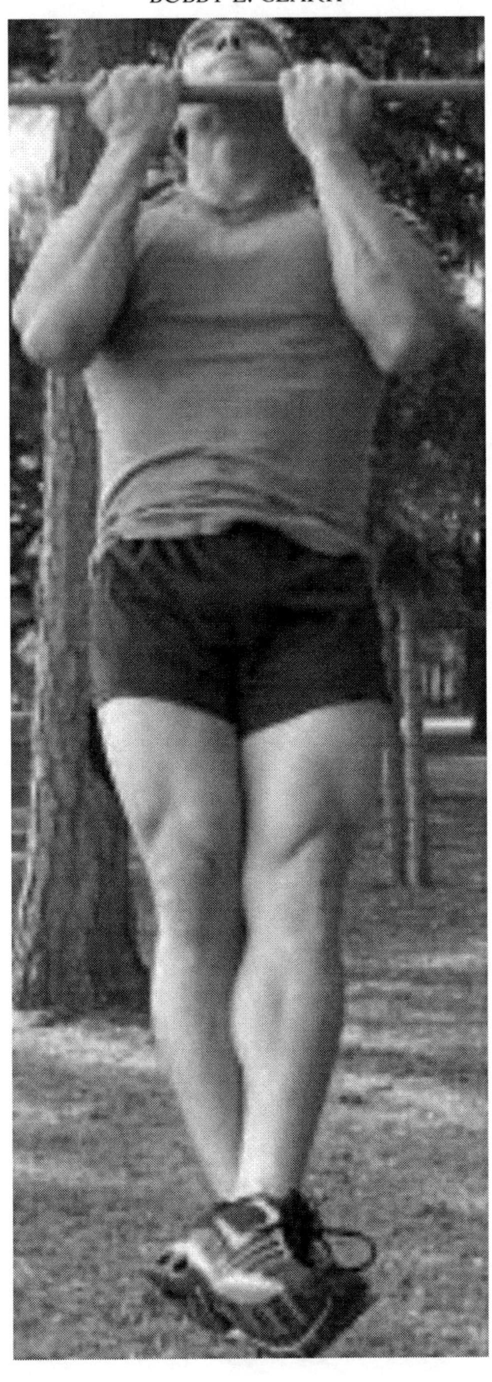

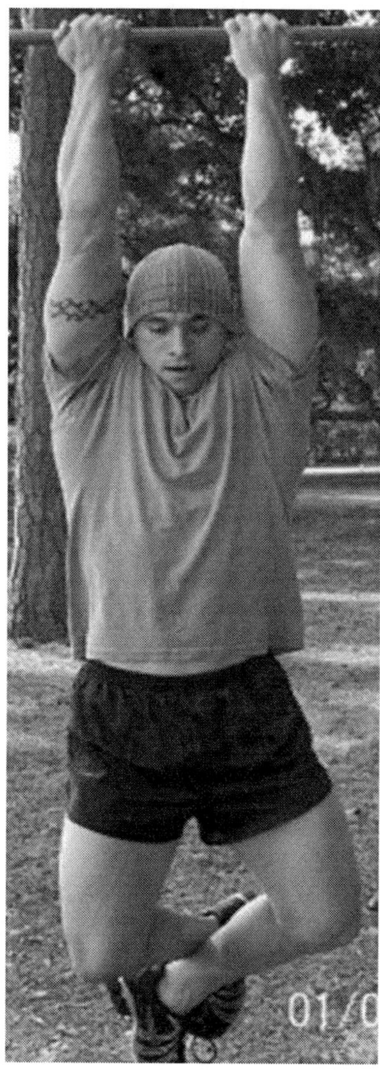

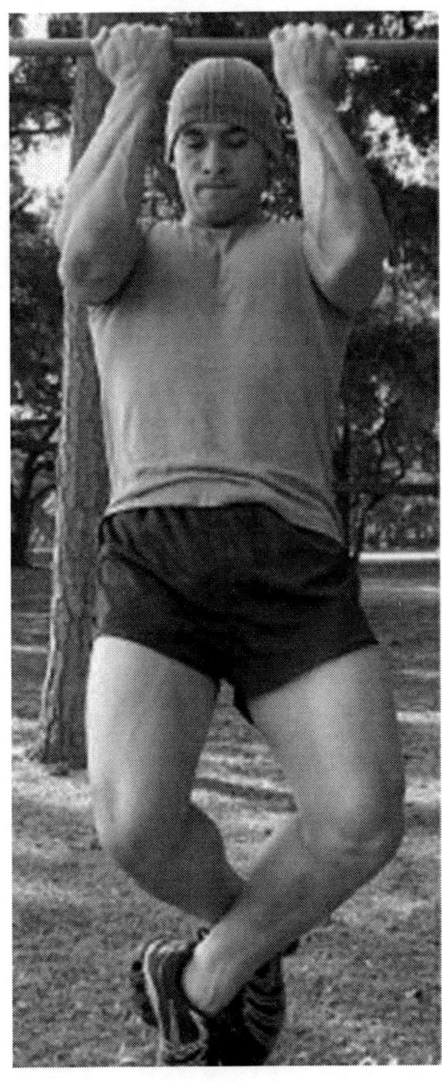

ONE ARM PULL-UPS: To begin with, there are very few people who can actually accomplish a true one arm pull-up. These pull-ups are adjusted so you can eventually build your way to a true one arm pull-up

STEPS:

1) Starting position for these bad boys are as follows. Take one hand and grasp the bar, palm towards you, thumb excluded. With the free hand grasp your wrist, palm facing you.
2) Now from a dead hang pull your chin to the bar, pause and descend. The key to developing strength in this exercise is in the hand grasping the wrist. You MUST attempt to use that arm as little as possible. By gradually decreasing the amount of use you will eventually get to the point of completing a true one arm pull-up.

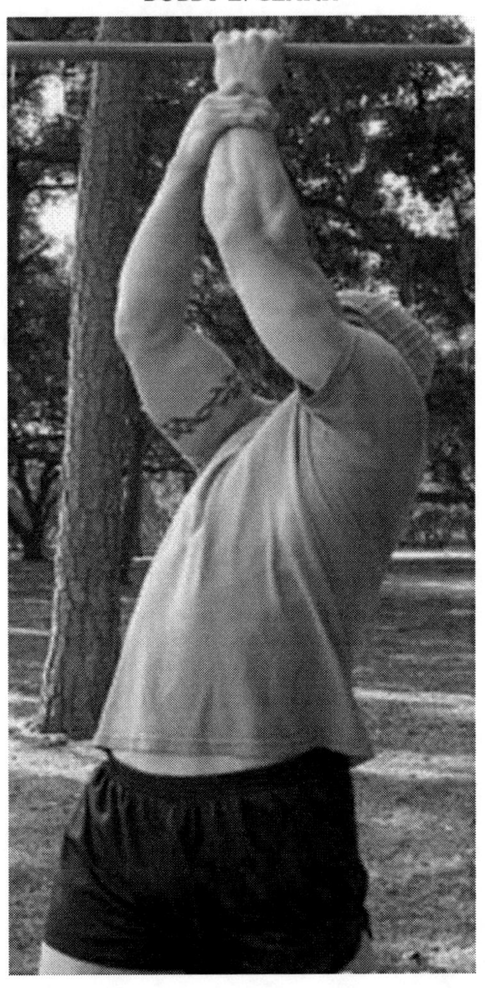

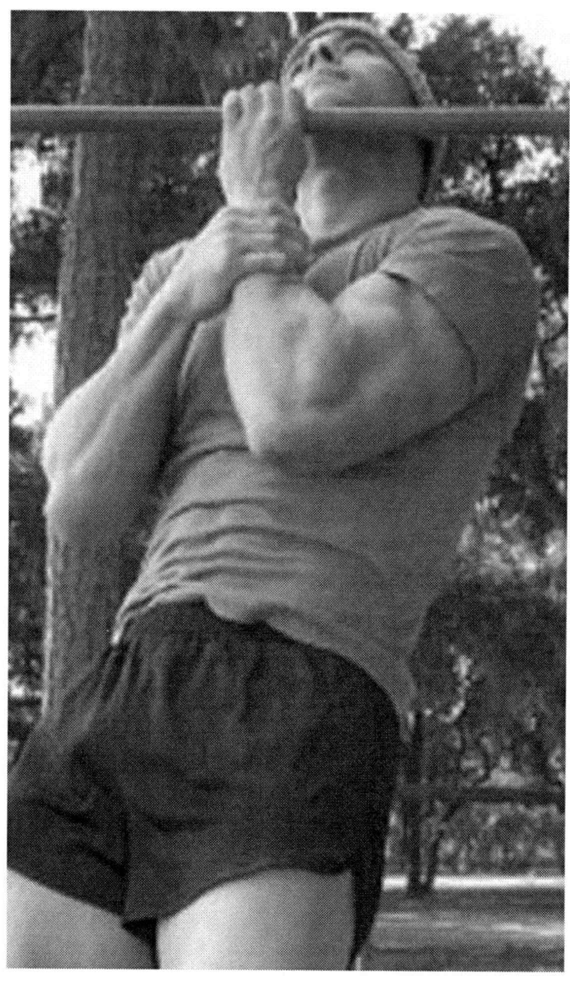

CHAPTER 3

TRICEPS

"Treat your body like a machine, quality fuel equals quality performance."

ONE ARM PUSH-UPS: Now any one can cheat their way through a one arm push-up, but where is the gain in that? Remember, quality before quantity, and you'll never have doubt in your training.

STEPS:

1) Okay, starting position is face down on the floor with your legs about two feet apart, and you should be on your toes. You should have one hand behind your back and the other hand fully extended supporting the weight of your body. A couple of key points: Insure your back stays straight, Resist the urge of allowing your hips to dip.
2) Now you're ready for rep one. Lower your CHEST down to the ground at a controlled pace, ensuring you keep your shoulders parallel to the ground. This will put maximum strain on your triceps.
4) Once at half rep (down) push back up for a rep of one. Once again resist the urge to dip and twist.

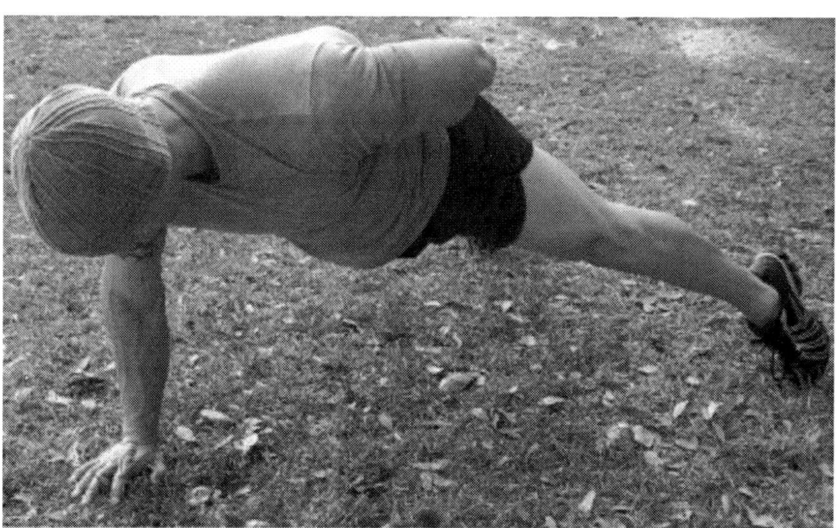

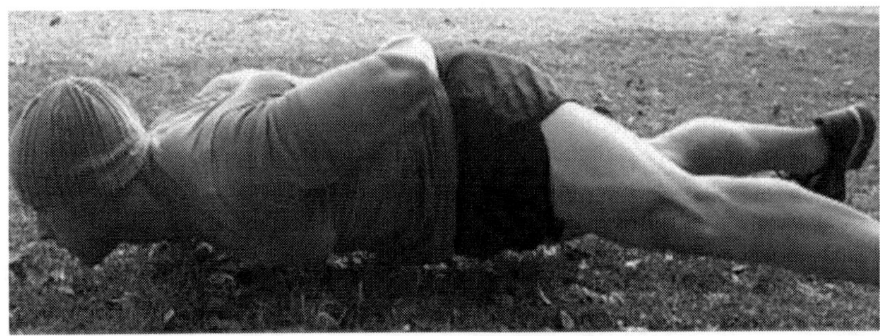

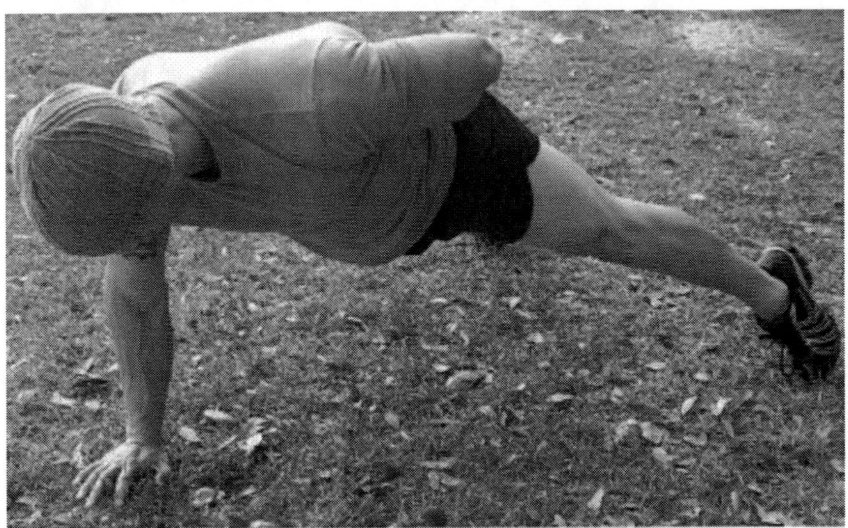

DIAMOND PUSH-UPS: Diamond push-ups are one of the more easily accomplished exercises, but these aren't your typical diamond push-ups.

STEPS:

1) Starting position should be this: Place index fingers and thumbs of each hand touching, forming a diamond shape between your hands. Your arms should be relaxed with your elbows tucked tightly to your sides, so your chest is resting on your hands. You should be on your toes as in most push-up positions.
2) Now from this position you will push-up utilizing your triceps to the half rep position (arms extended), next rock back on your toes until your hands are directly in front of your face.
3) You are still at half rep, now lower your body down until your nose touches the ground between your hands. As you lower your body down, you ensure that your elbows are tucked in tight and your hands stay flat on the ground. This will ensure isolation of the triceps.
4) From here you simply rock forward on your toes until your hands are once again resting under your chest, and you are back in the starting position. Remember, you should not lie on your hands, and support the weight of your body with your triceps. Feel the burn, and don't cheat.

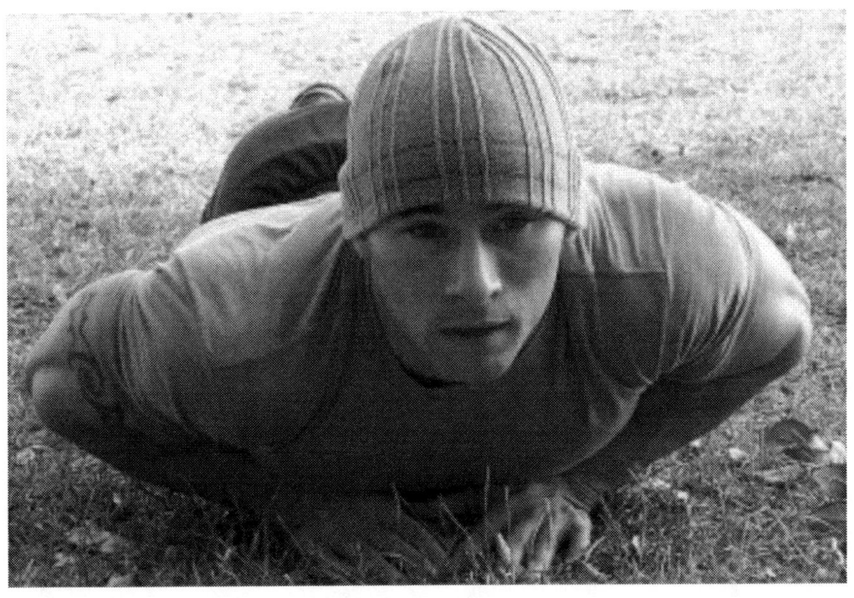

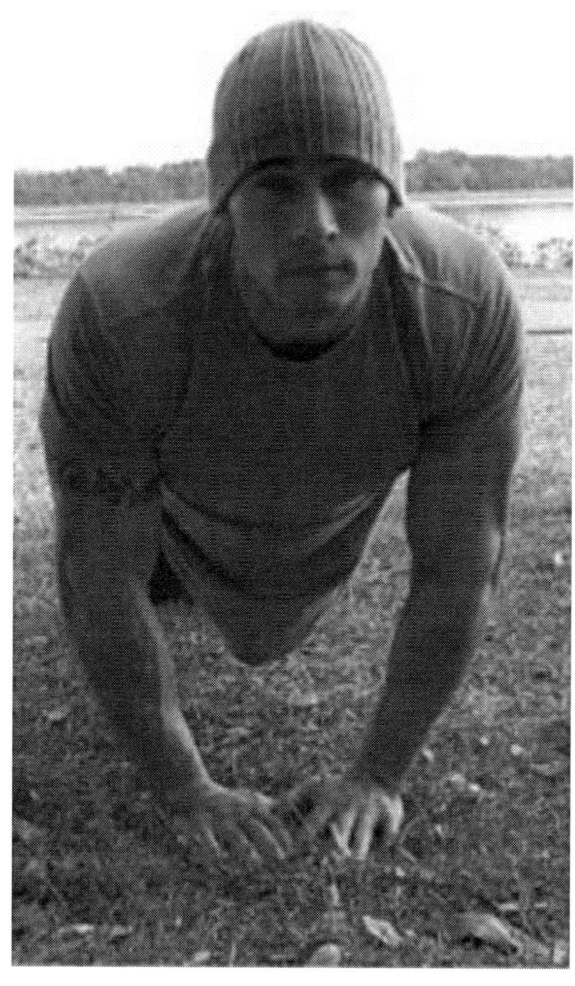

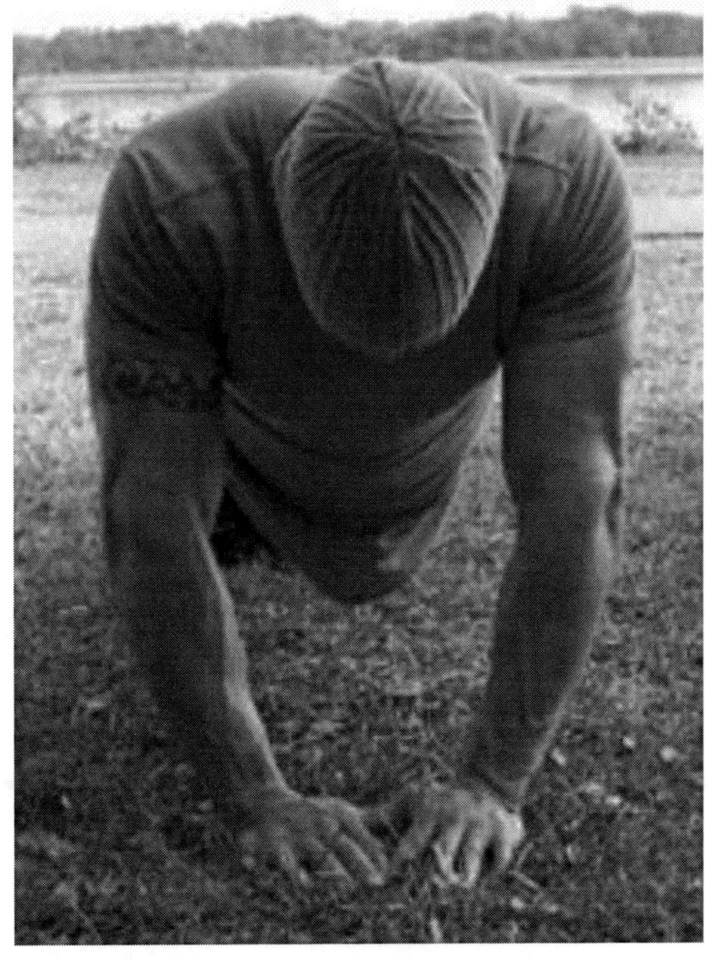

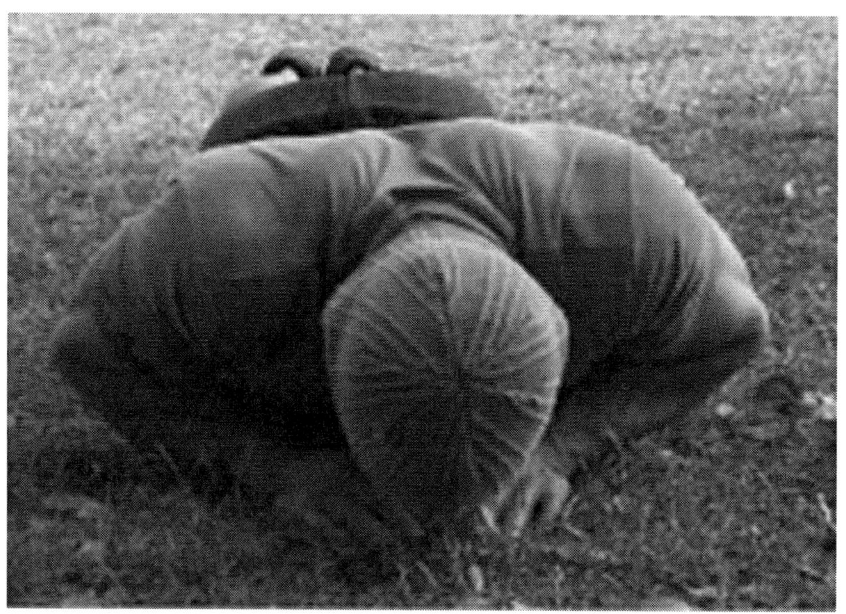

HAMMER PUSH-UPS: The only thing you need for this exercise is a stair step, a curb, or anything that can give you around eight to ten inches of clearance.

STEPS:

1) Begin by placing your hands together as if you were going to pray. Now make fists with your hands so they are knuckle-to-knuckle and heel-to-heel.
2) Next place your hands as if they were on the edge of the step or curb. From this position, you make an upside down "V" with your body. Ensure that you are on your toes. This is your starting position.
3) Now slowly lower your body down towards your hands by allowing only your elbows to bend (keep your elbows in tight to your body). Your head should slide between your arms putting the majority of your body weight on your triceps as you descend. Be careful not to allow your head to hit the ground. Once your head is close to the ground, stop as you are at half rep.
4) From here explode up with your triceps, pressing your body back into the starting position. Now rep them out and build those triceps.

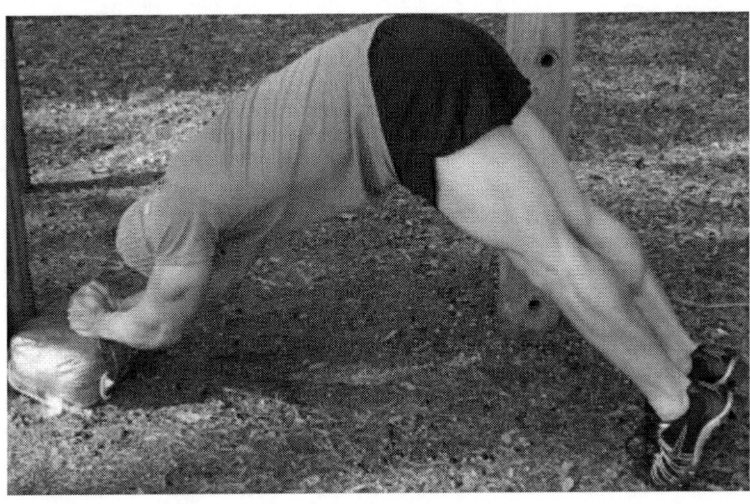

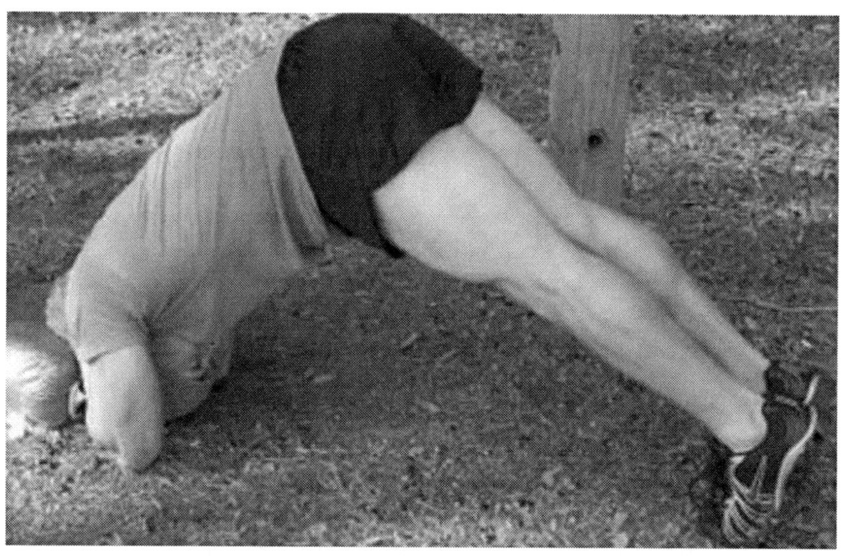

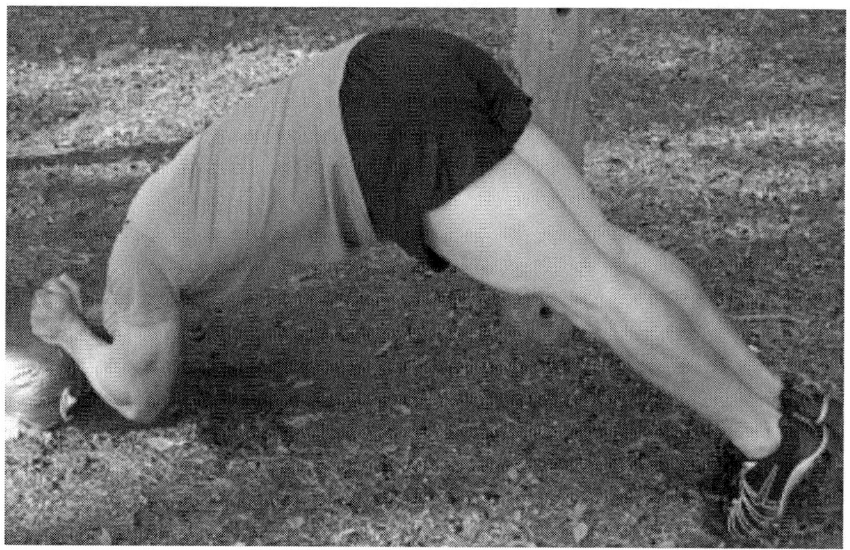

HIGH AND TIGHTS: High and tights are yet another exercise you can do anywhere to get a great pump to your triceps.

STEPS:

1) First place your hands on the ground as you would for a diamond push-up.
2) From this position, you extend your arms and make that inverted "V" with your body as you do in the Hindu push-ups.
3) Now from here, simply lower your nose down to your hands at a controlled pace. Once your nose has reached your hands, you pause for a one count. (Ensure you do not rest directly on your hands).
4) Finally, exhale and press your body back to the starting position (arms fully extended). That's rep one. Now shred them up!

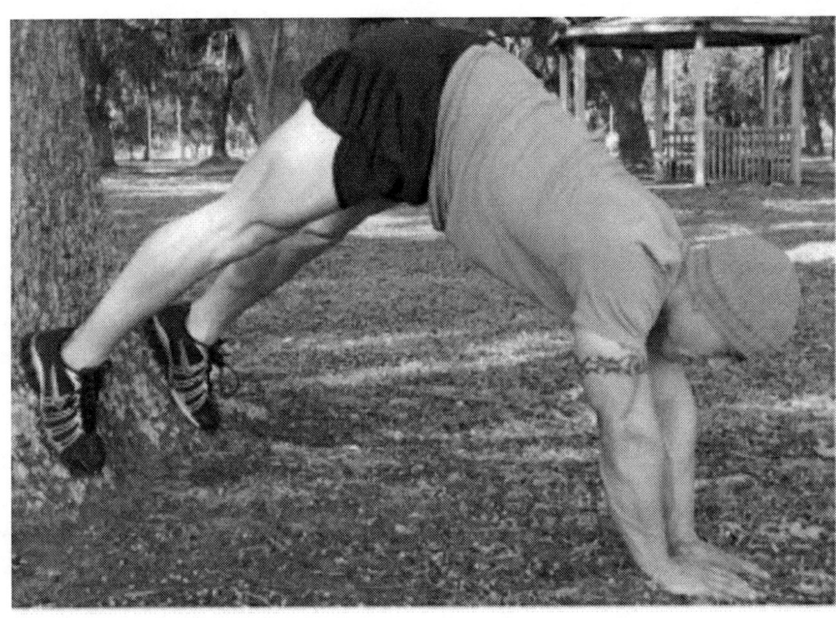

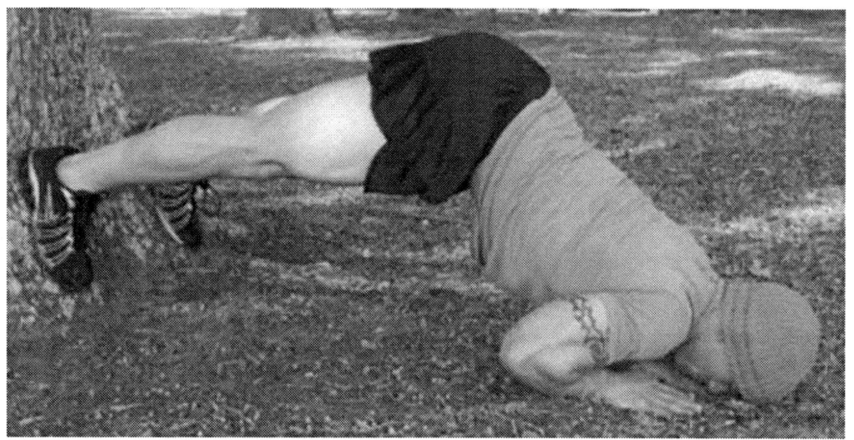

CHAPTER 4

BACK

"Your willpower will give out way before your muscles do. Just remember; it's all in your mind."

GORILLAS: This exercise rocks for developing those lower traps and inner lats, not to mention a killer abdominal workout.

STEPS:

1) First mount the bar in a pull-up position (palms away) with your grip just outside the width of your shoulders. This is your starting position.
3) Now with as little momentum as possible, you raise your shins to the bar while simultaneously pulling your body to the bar. Once you've reached the bar with your hips, you hold this position for a one count by squeezing your back as if you were trying to touch your elbows behind your back.
4) Let's get to it. Next slowly lower yourself back down to the starting position. If this exercise is too difficult for you to accomplish, simple do the exercise with bent knees rather than straight legs.

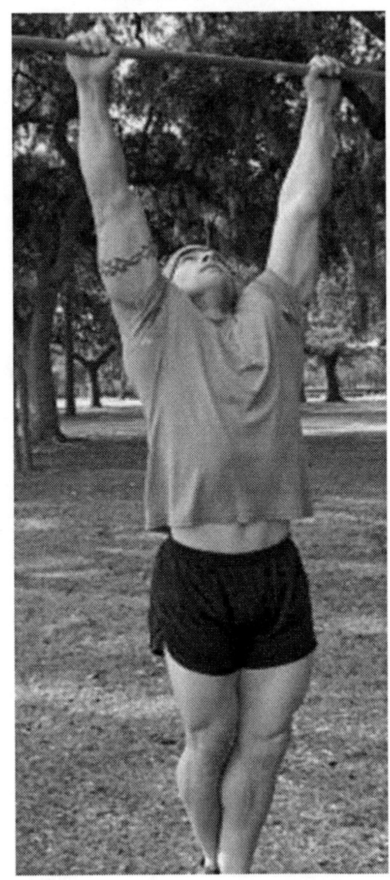

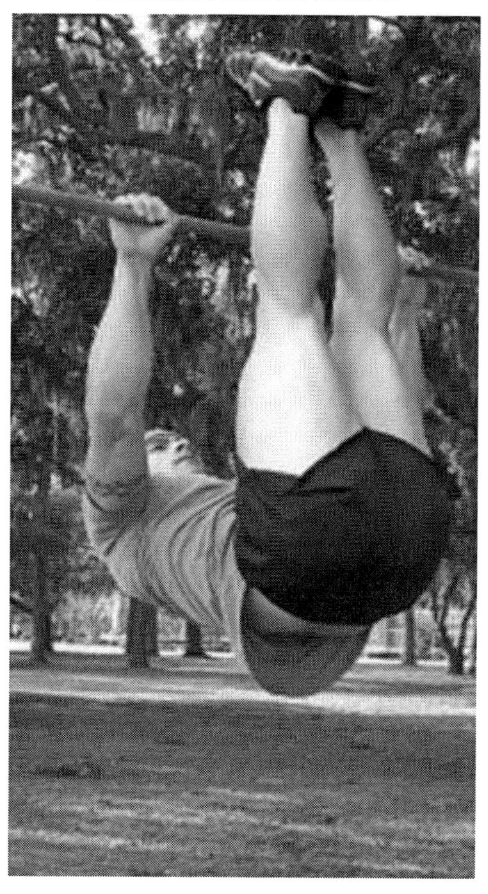

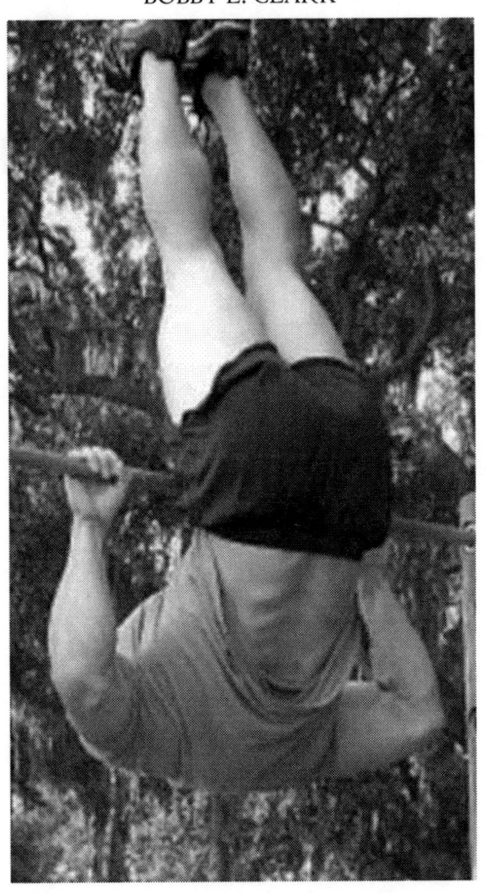

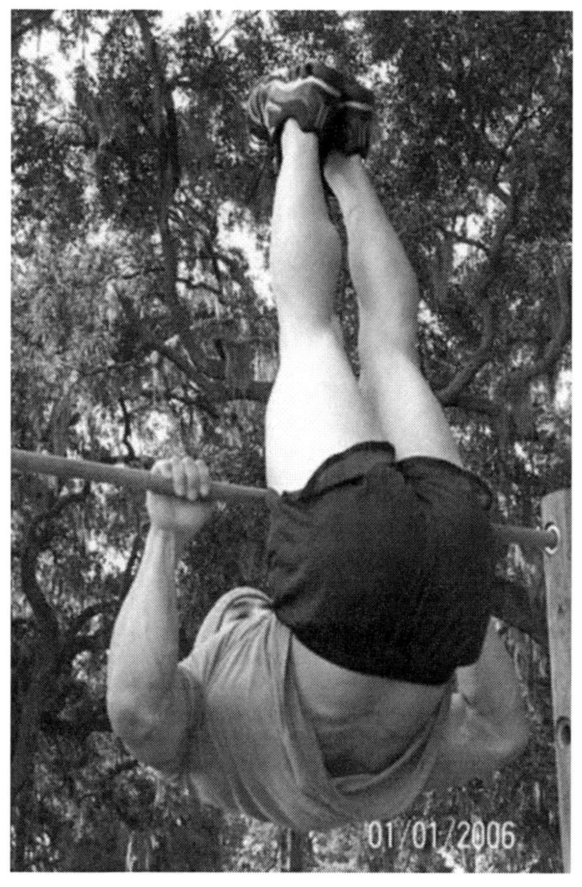
01/01/2006

PULL-UPS: Pull-ups are one of the oldest and most accessible exercises around, yet so many people lack the upper body strength to accomplish just one. In this section I am going to show you two different variations of the typical pull-up that will catapult your strength and size.

VARIATION ONE "1-3-5" COUNT PULL-UPS:

STEPS:

1) Okay, mount the bar in the pull-up position and come to a dead hang. Now remember it's all in the count. In a one second count, roll your shoulders back, then pause.
2) Now pull up until your chin is above the bar. You must now hold this position for a count of three seconds.
3) Once you've reached three, slowly lower your bodies by relaxing your back at a five count pace. That's one rep.

NOTE: Ensure when you pull up, you pull straight up as if your nose had to follow an imaginary rope hanging from the center of the pull up bar. By doing so you will isolate the lats.

VARIATION TWO CHEST PULL-UPS: This is awesome for getting a full peak flex out of those lats and lower traps (trapezoids).

STEPS:

1) Once again mount the bar. Come to a dead hang.
2) Now at a one-count pace, pull your lower chest to the bar.
3) Hold this position for one count; you concentrate on squeezing your back in tight. Try to touch your elbows together behind your back.
4) Now simply lower your body down by slowly relaxing your back at the bottom to ensure you feel that good stretch.

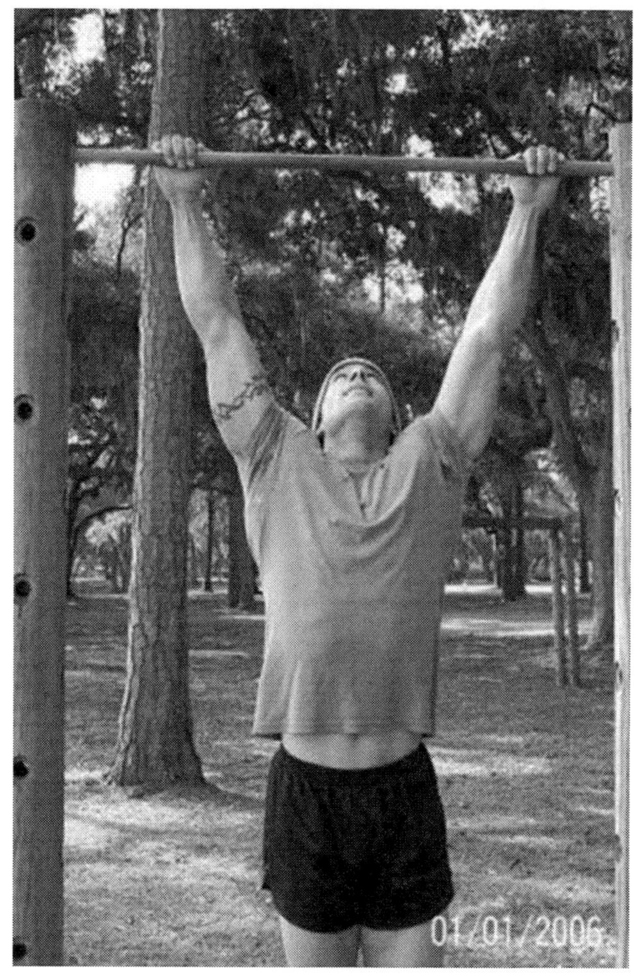
01/01/2006

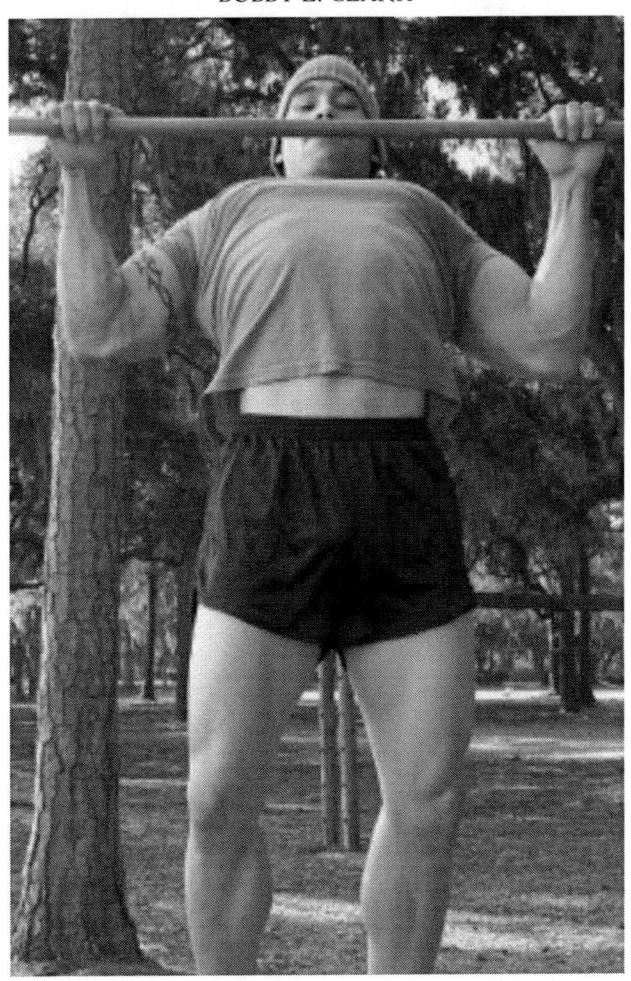

INVERTED LEG LIFTS: One area of the back that is often neglected, though detrimental to a truly strong physique, is the lower back. Most back injuries are lower lumbar injuries due to week muscles under heavy strain. So how do you develop it? Simple, find yourself a wall.

STEPS:

1) Now begin in a headstand position with your back to the wall. This is the starting position.
2) Now slowly lower your straight legs down until they are parallel to the ground. Pause for a count of one.
3) Now simply return to the starting position by raising your legs back up. These are not as easy as they look. You'll see. If these are too difficult for you to do or pose too much strain on your back, simply do the exercise with bent knees.

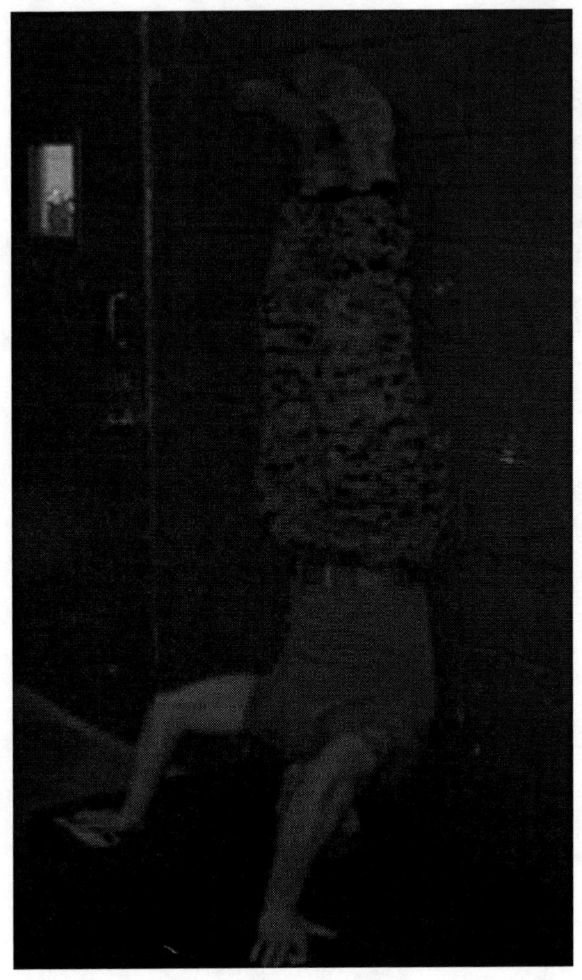

UNLEASH THE MACHINE

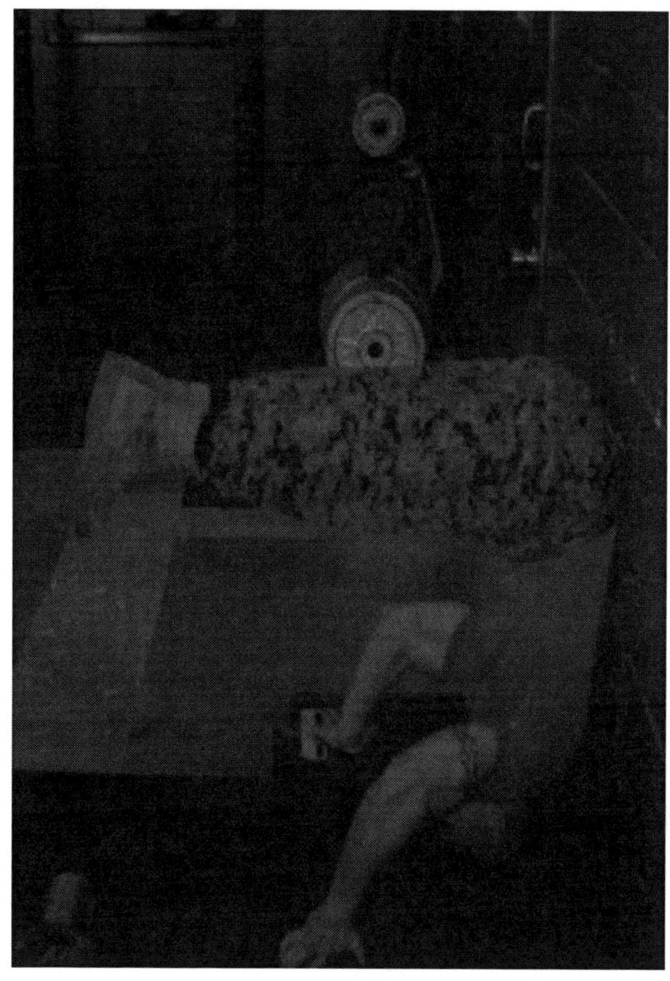

CHAPTER 5

CHEST

"Ninety percent of difficult training is mental; therefore, a weak-minded person will inevitably be, just weak."

BUDDY PUSH-UPS: This is one of the few exercises that you will need a partner for. So find yourself a buddy and prepare to really work.

STEPS:

1) Begin by taking a typical push-up position (chest on the ground, hand on the ground near your chest, either close or wide grip, and head looking straight forward).
2) Now have your partner stand at your head at least two or three feet away.
3) Next have your partner place both of their palms on the top center or your shoulders (just below the large cervical vertebrae at the base of your neck).
4) Your partner should place as much of his/her body weight on their hands as you can handle.
5) From this position, simply push up, as you would do in ordinary push-ups (don't be disappointed if you only get a few).
6) Now that you are the top of rep one, hold for a one count while squeezing your chest.
7) Next, return to the original starting position. DO NOT LET your body rest on the ground. Pause for one count, then continue. I bet you never though a push-up could be so tough.

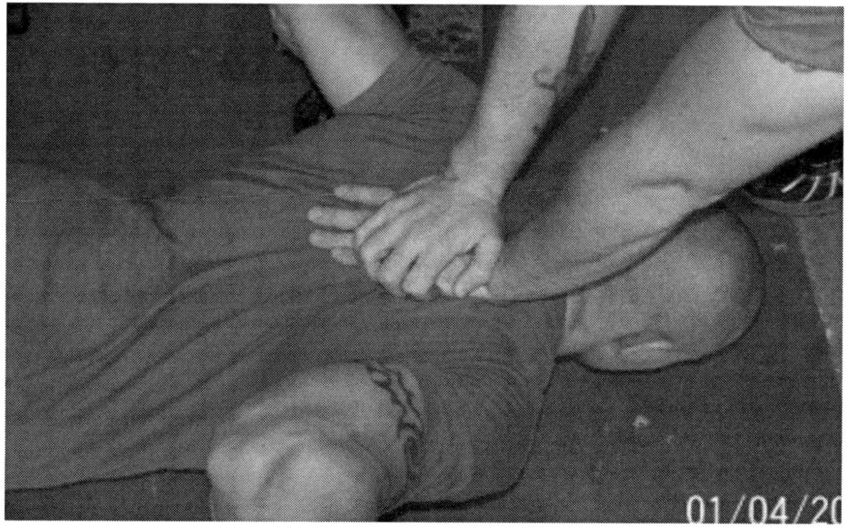

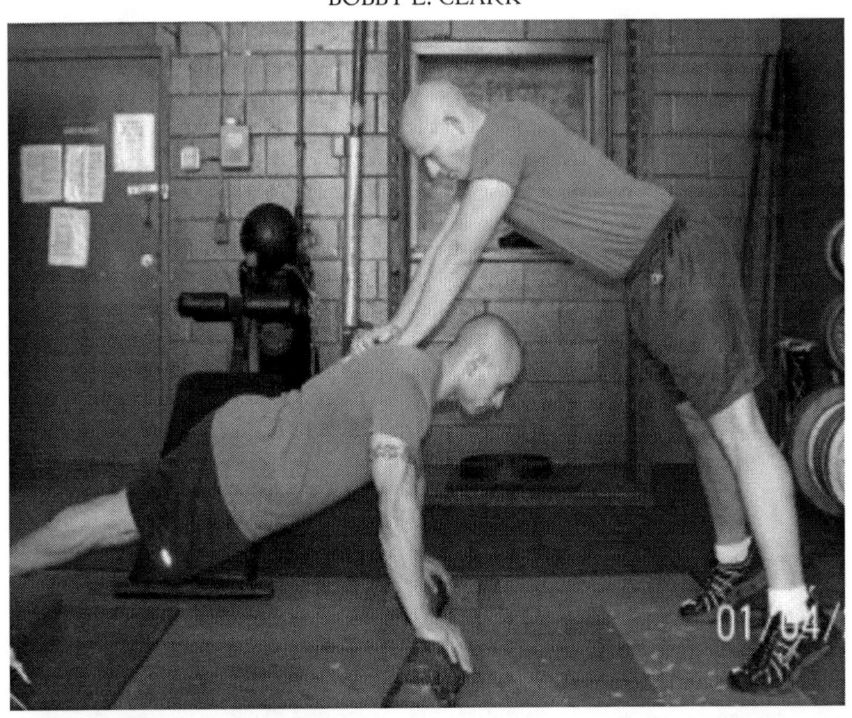
01/04/

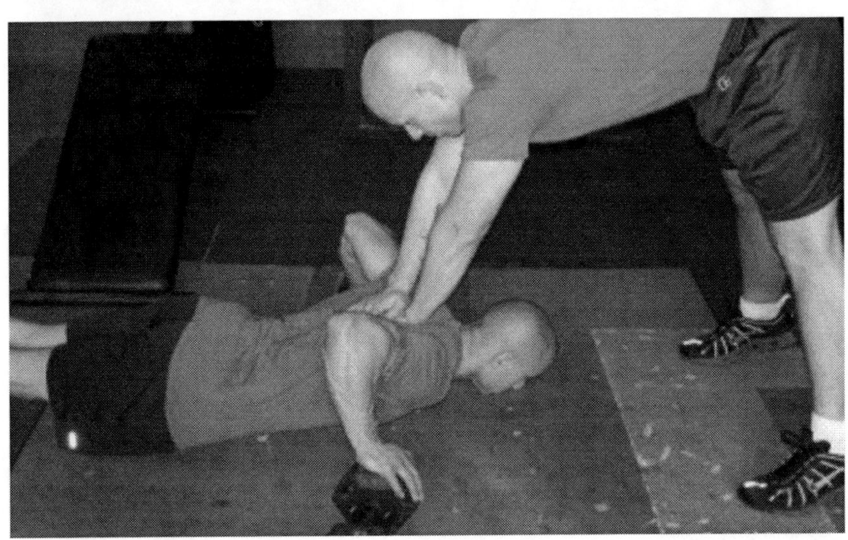

BALISTIC PUSH-UPS: These are great for developing a powerful chest and can be done either with your feet on the ground, or elevated. The only things you need for this exercise are two objects to elevate your hands at least eight inches from the ground. You can use books, bricks, or even sandbags. For this exercise I use sandbags.

STEPS:

1) Start in the normal push-up position (chest on the ground) with your hands in the neutral position. You should have the "sandbags" placed just to the outside of your hands.
2) From here explode off the ground by pressing your body up so your hands leave the ground.
3) As you come down, move your hands outward so they land on the sandbags.
4) Now lower your body back down as far as you can (this part of the exercise is controlled, not explosive).
5) Once at the bottom of this movement, explode back up so that your hands leave the sandbags. As your body comes down, bring your hands back to the inside of the sandbags and lower your body back down to the starting position. That's one rep, now let's keep the sweat flowing and pump out as many as we can.

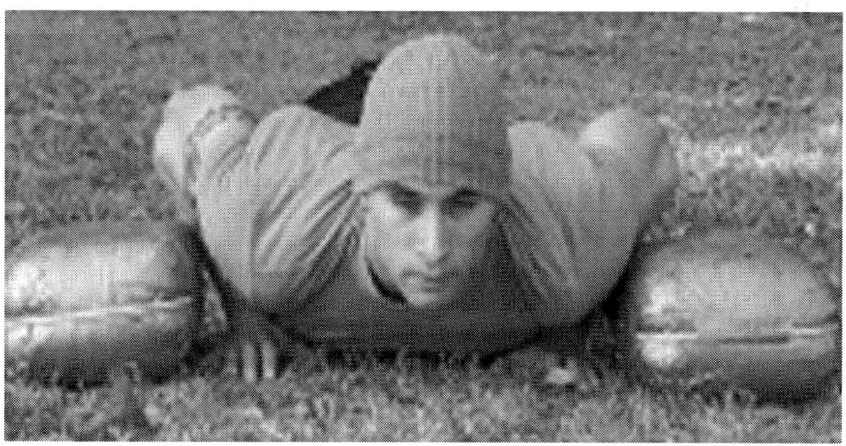

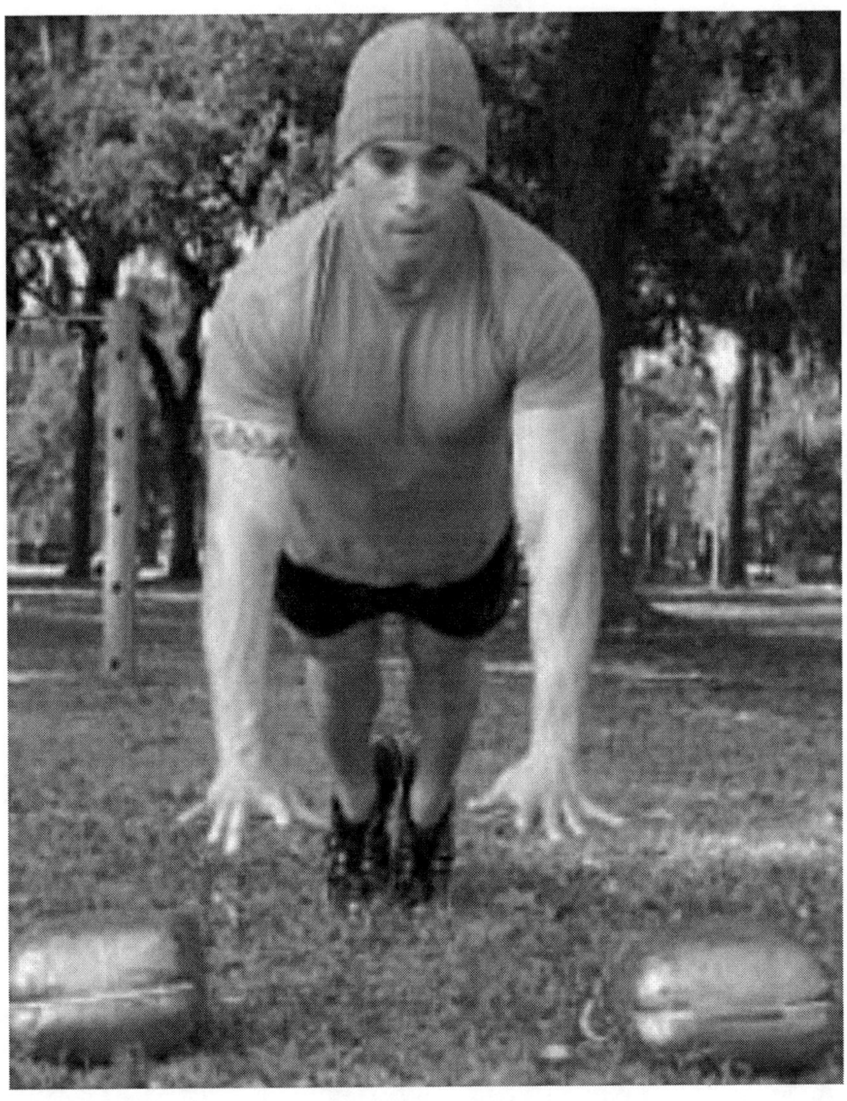

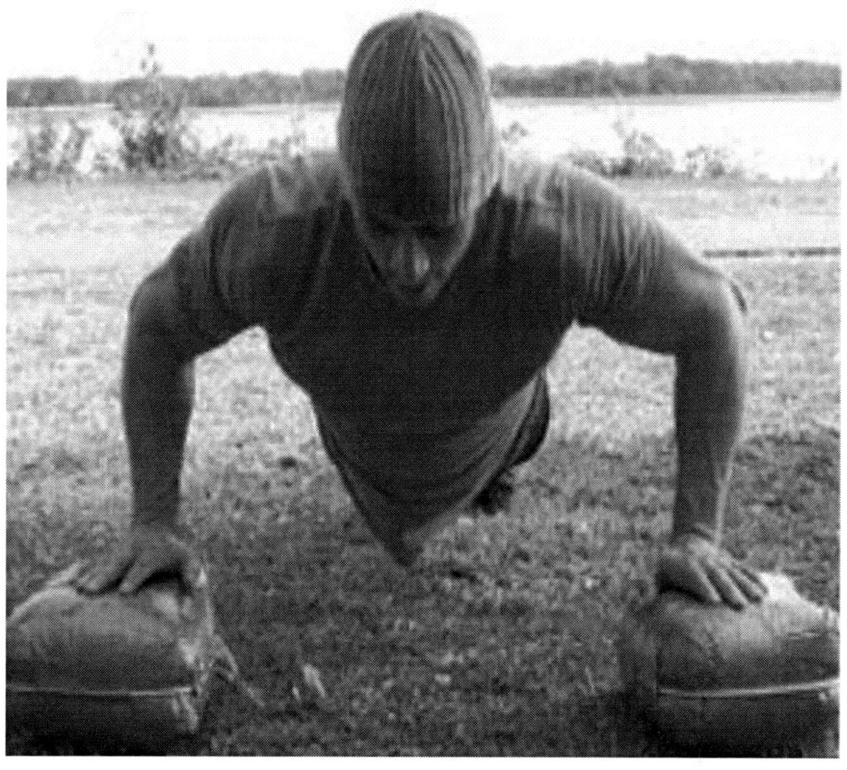

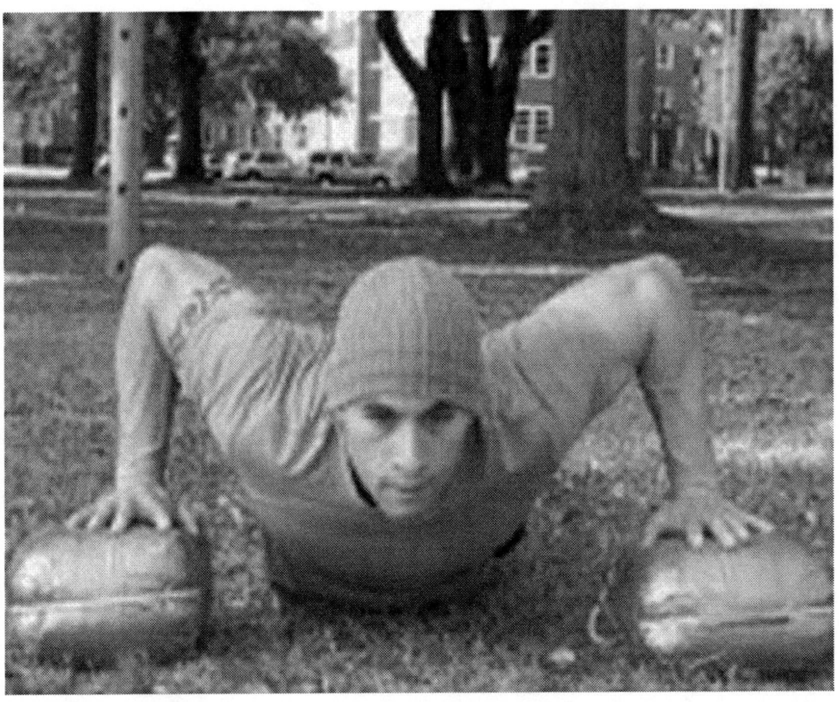

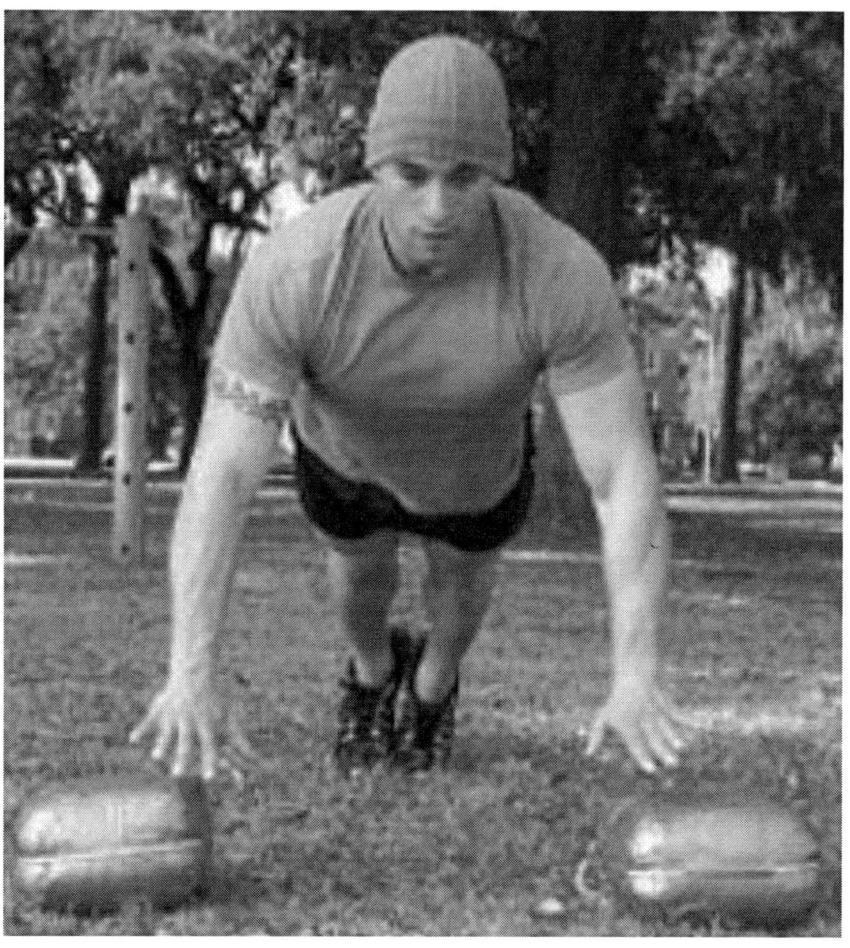

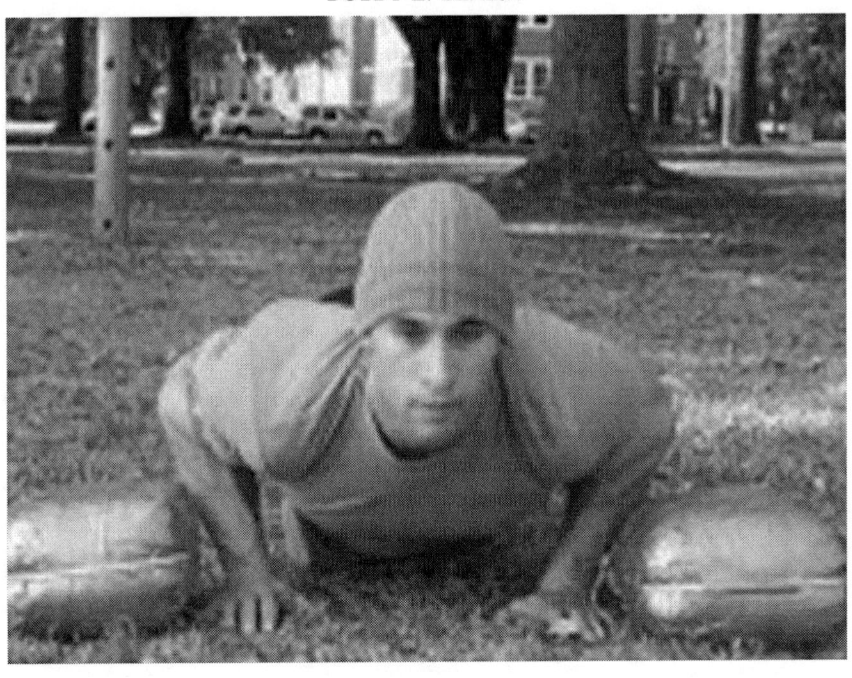

ALTERNATING PUSH-UPS: These are awesome for stretching and building the inner portion of your chest. Once again you will need something to elevate your hands. I again chose a sandbag.

STEPS:

1) Starting position is once again the typical push-up position, with a couple variations.
2) Your hand width is neutral with one palm on the ground and the other palm on top of the sandbag that is positioned by your side.
3) Next explode by pressing your body up and over with the hand that is on the sandbag. While you are in the air, alternate the hand is on the sandbag.
4) So...as you come down, the hand that was previously on the sandbag should now be on the ground, and your body should be on the other side of the sandbag.
5) You must ensure that your feet stay on the ground and act as a pivot points. This is easily accomplished by crossing your feet so that only one foot is on the ground.

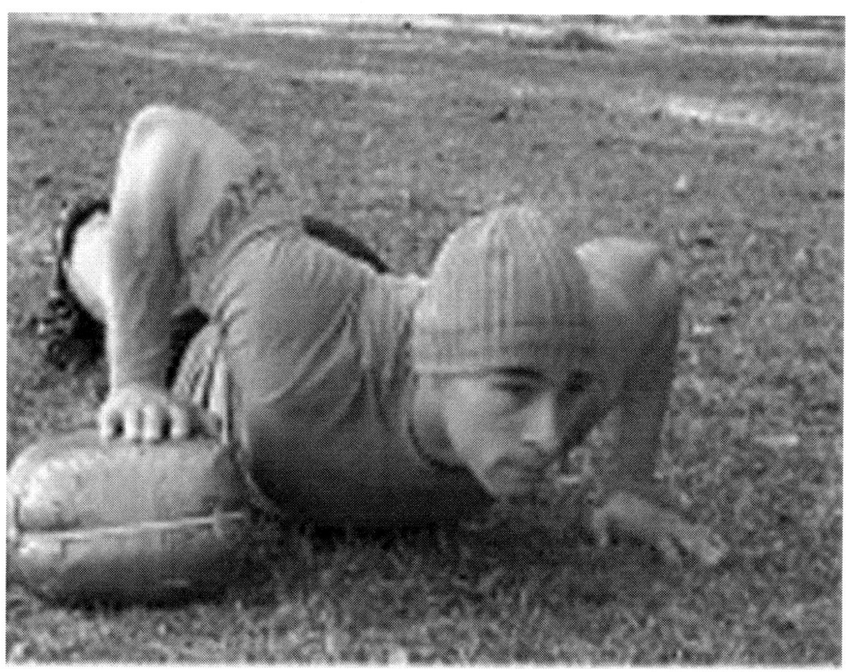

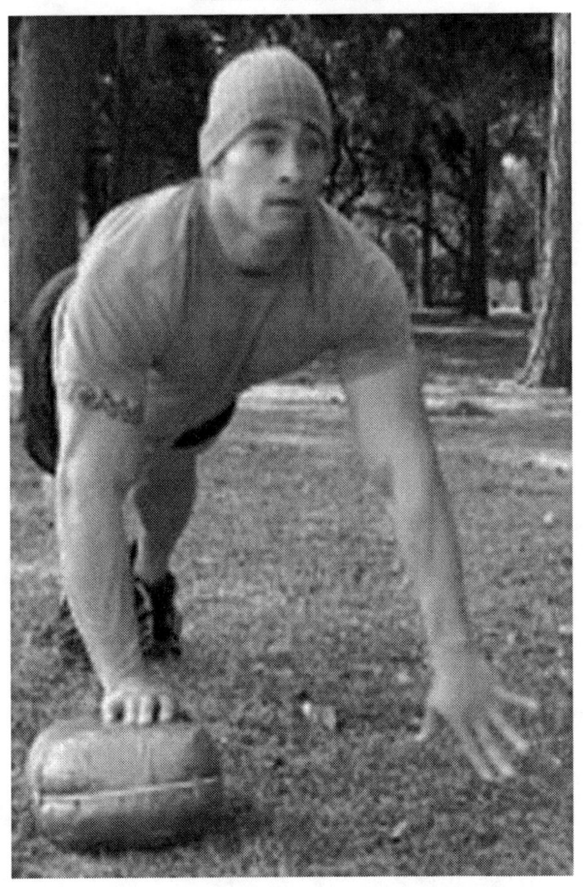

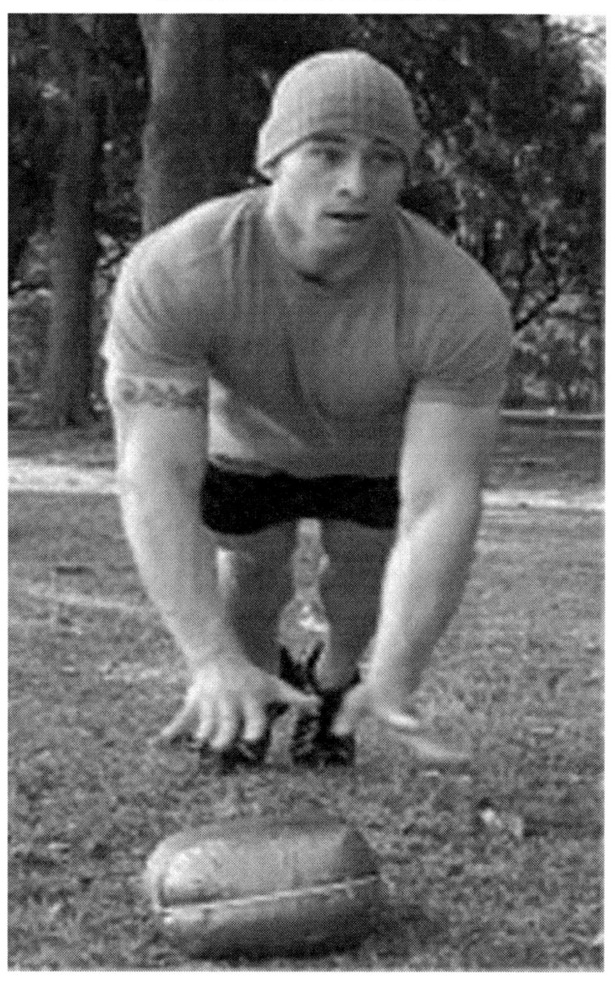

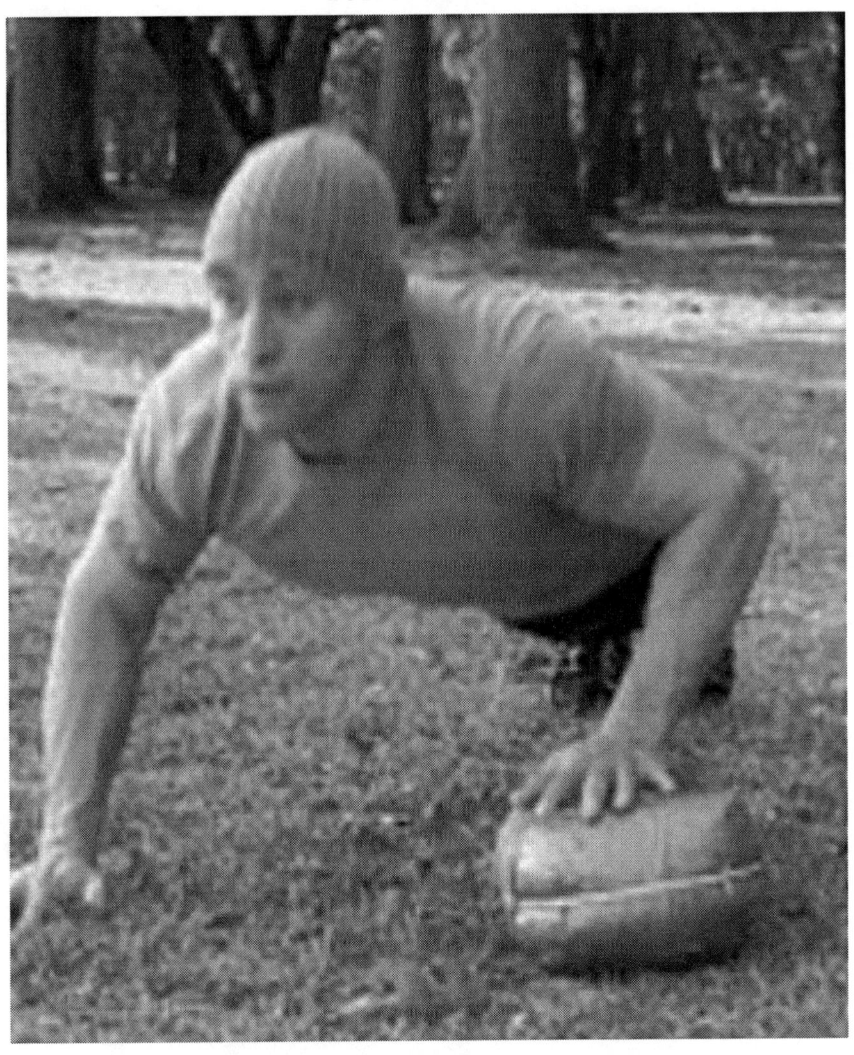

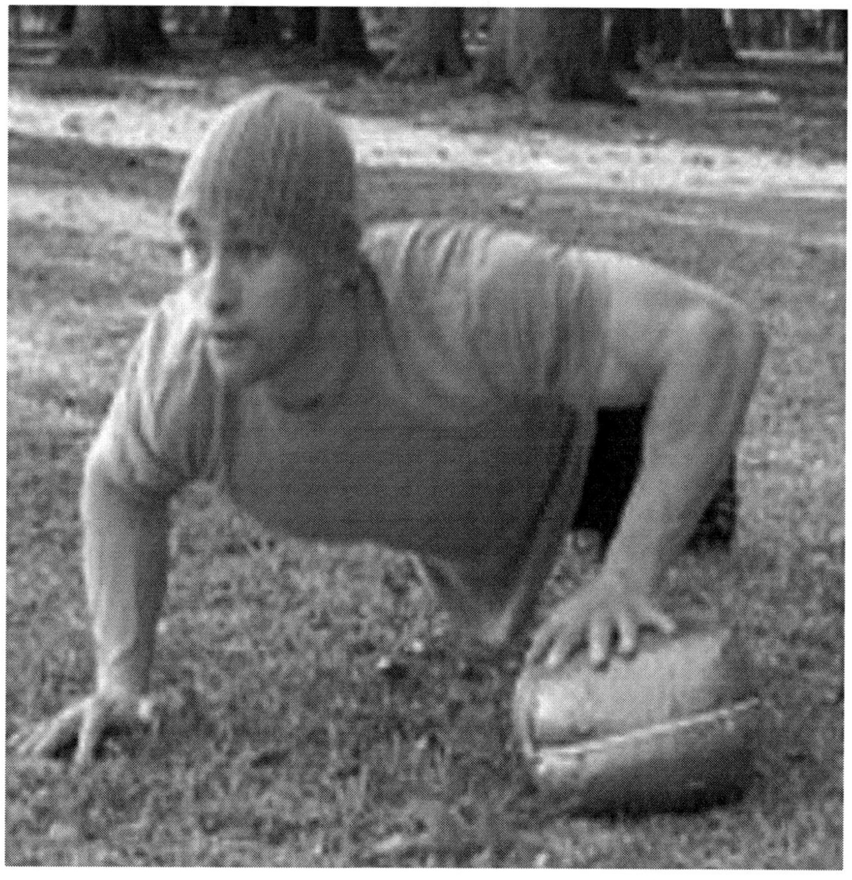

PERPENDICULAR PUSH-UPS: These are awesome for isolating and developing muscularity to your whole chest.

STEPS:

1) Begin in the normal push-up position except with your arms extended and positioned slightly wider that your shoulders.
2) Now take your hands and turn them out so your fingertips point away from each other as if they were on an imaginary line running perpendicular to your body's centerline.
3) Next rock forward on your toes, attempting to put one hundred percent of your body weight on your hands (your feet should only be used for balance).
4) Now, keeping your head up and looking forward, slowly lower your body down until your chest is just above the ground.
5) Pause for one count, then press your body back into the starting position. That's one rep. Keep it up!

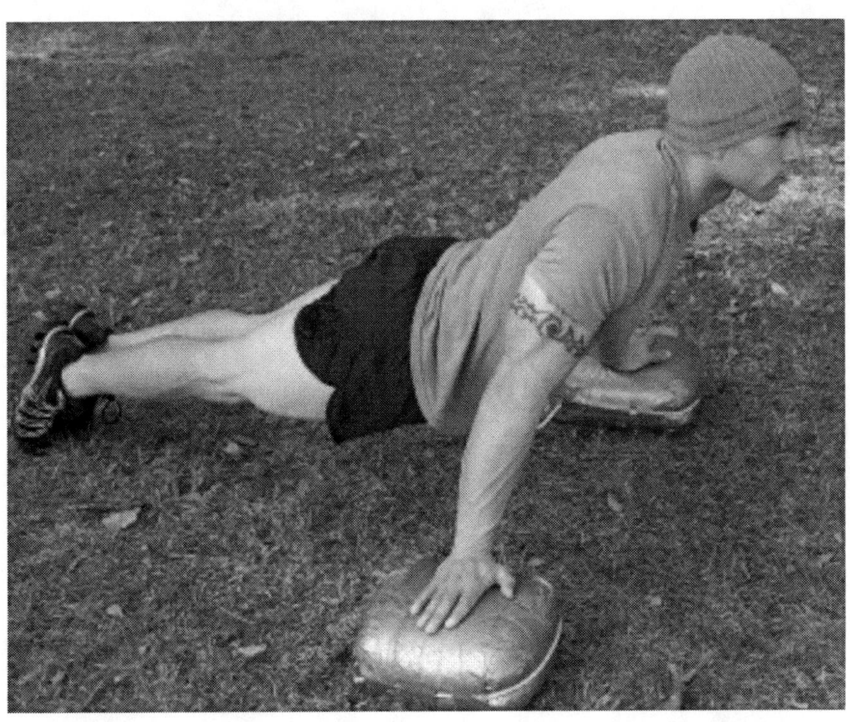

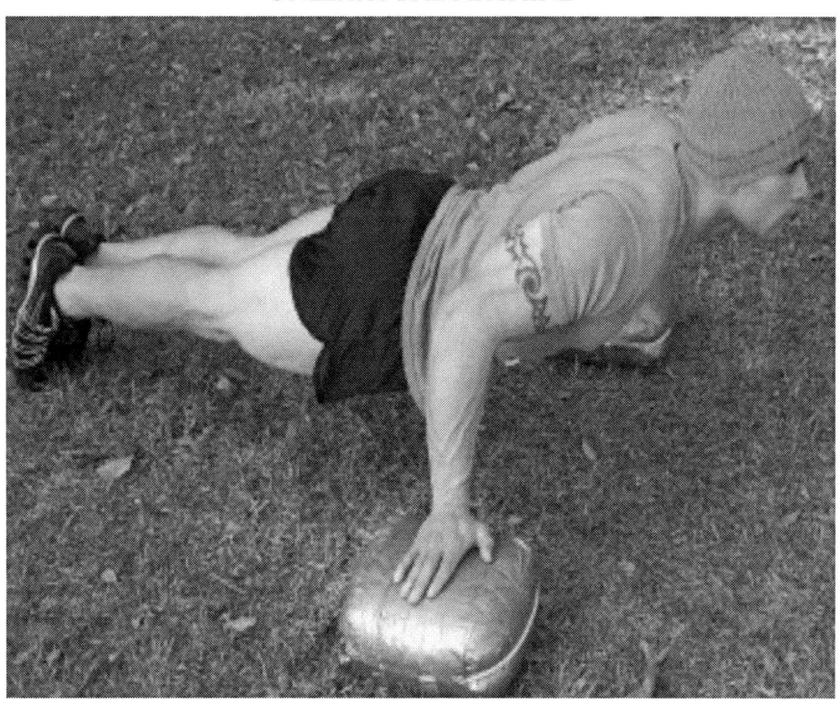

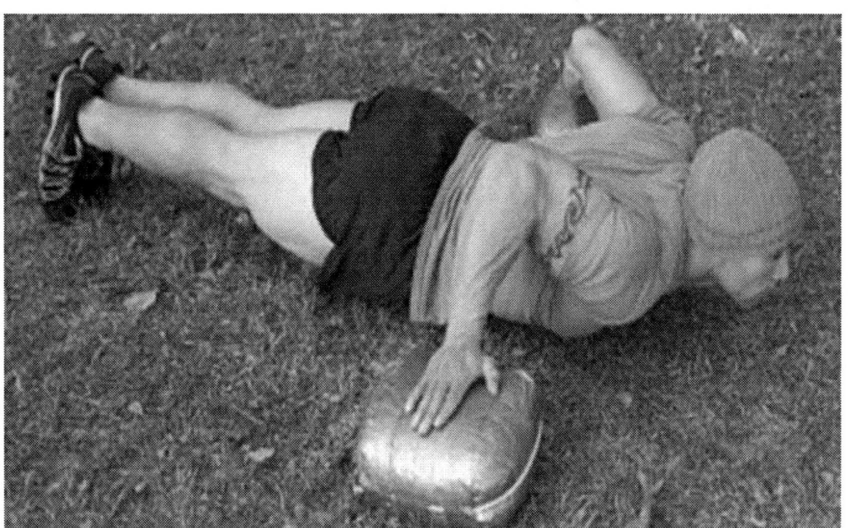

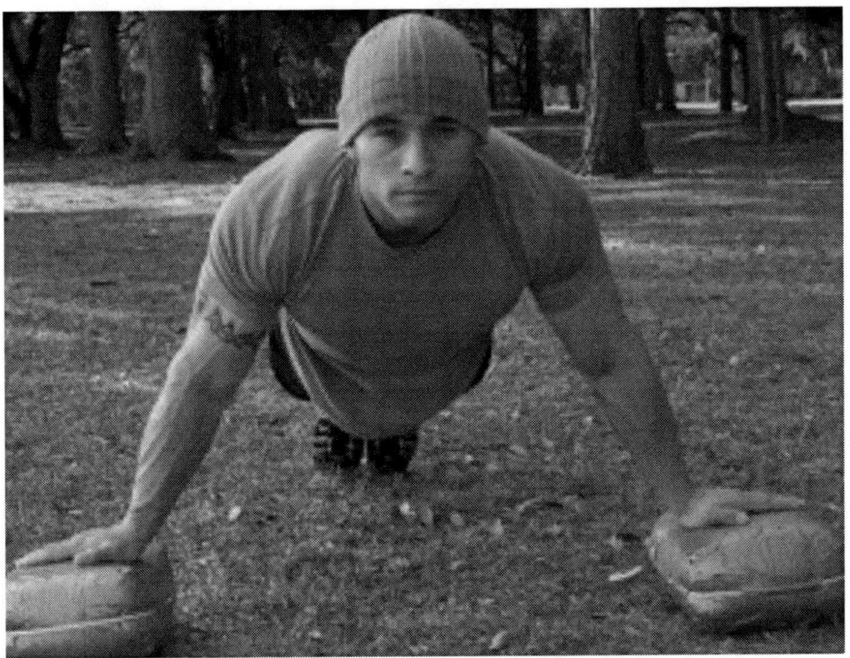

A LITTLE MORE: The best way to develop your chest is to elevate your hands by using something like the sandbags you see me using. I made these by filling two bags with sand and packing them so there is no space left in the bag. Next wrap it in a trash bag to seal it. Then I simply take a roll of duct tape and go to town. The elevation works so well because it enables you to get a deeper stretch.

CHAPTER 6

LEGS

"You are only limited by your level of determination."

ONE LEGGED SQUATS: You thought squatting a few hundred pounds on the squat rack was tough. Give this a try.

STEPS:

1) Start by raising your arms out to your sides or in front of you for balance.
2) Now raise one of your legs about waist high.
3) Next slowly lower your body down, ensuring your foot stays flat on the ground and you don't go too fast.
4) Once your butt has touched your foot, pause for a one count. Now raise you body back up. Now that's a work out!

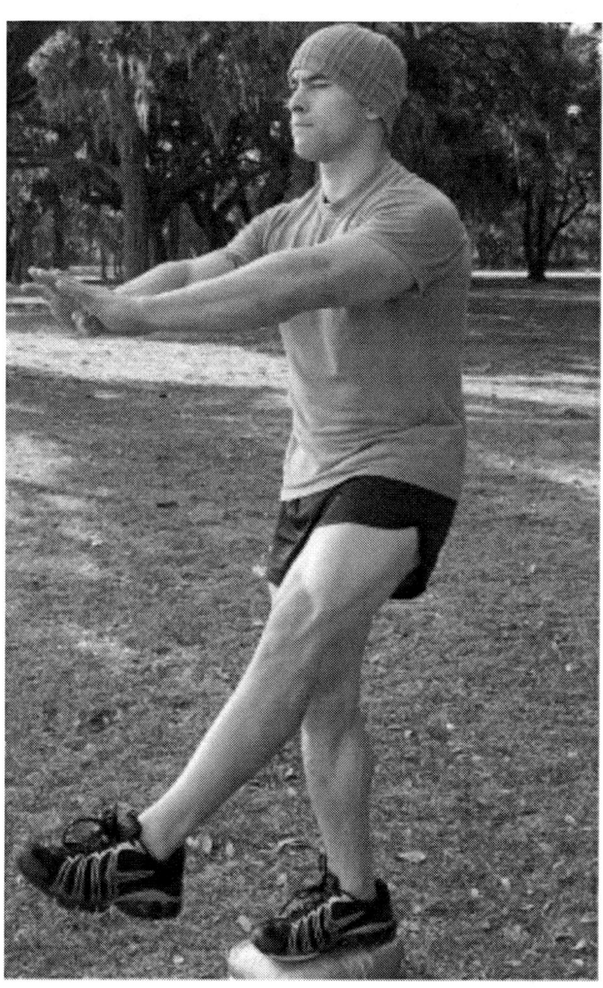

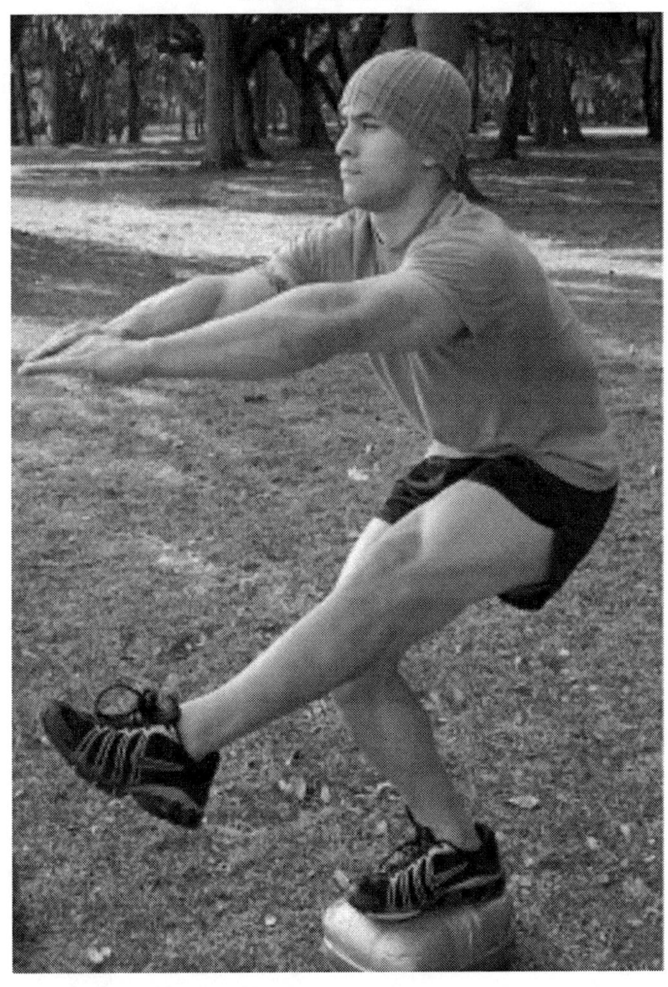

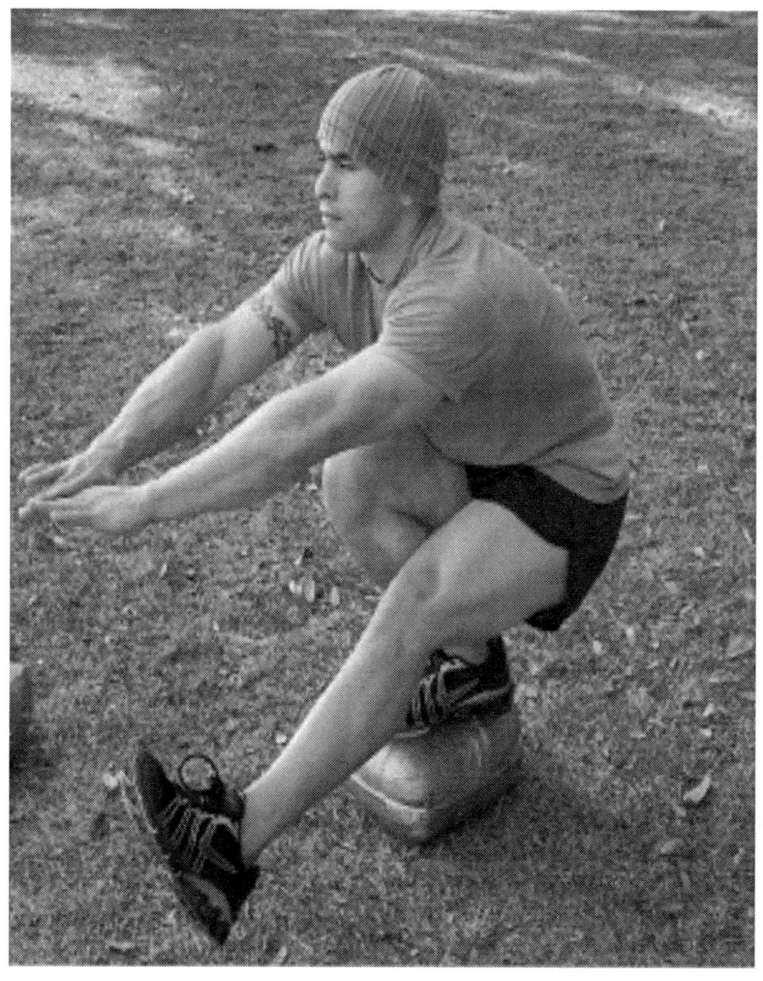

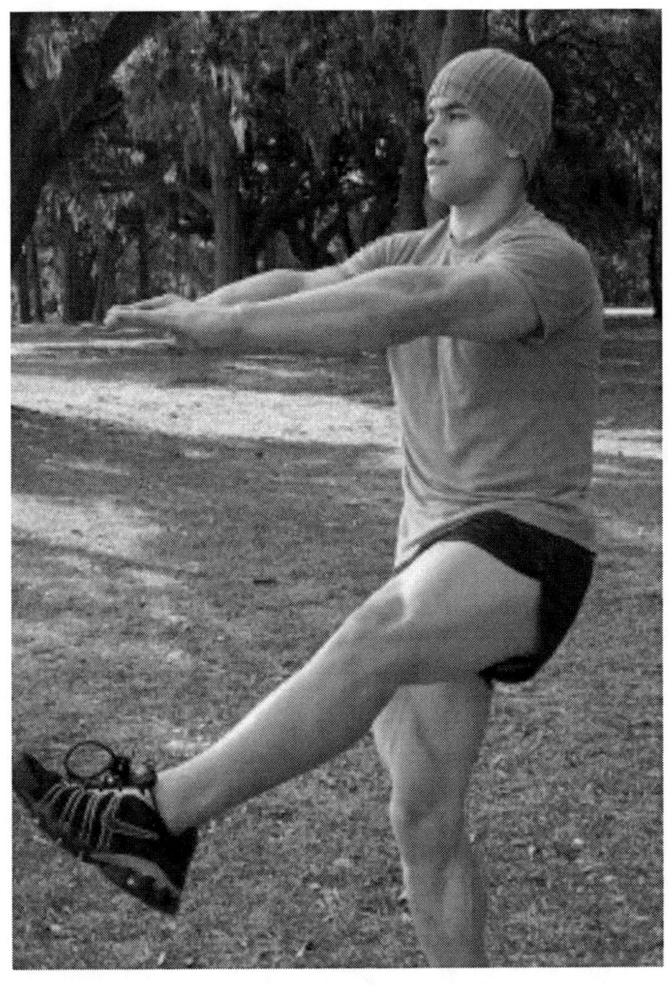

HINDU SQUATS: These are more of an endurance exercise that always gets an awesome burn in both your legs and your lungs.

<u>STEPS:</u>

1) Start with your feet about shoulder width apart and your hands behind your back.
3) Ensuring you keep your back straight bend at the knees, lower your body down until your butt touches your heels.
4) Pause briefly, then stand back up at a controlled rate simultaneously bringing your hands to your front.
5) Once you are completely standing flex your quadriceps and gluts for a one count while you bring your hands behind your back. That's one rep now pump them out.

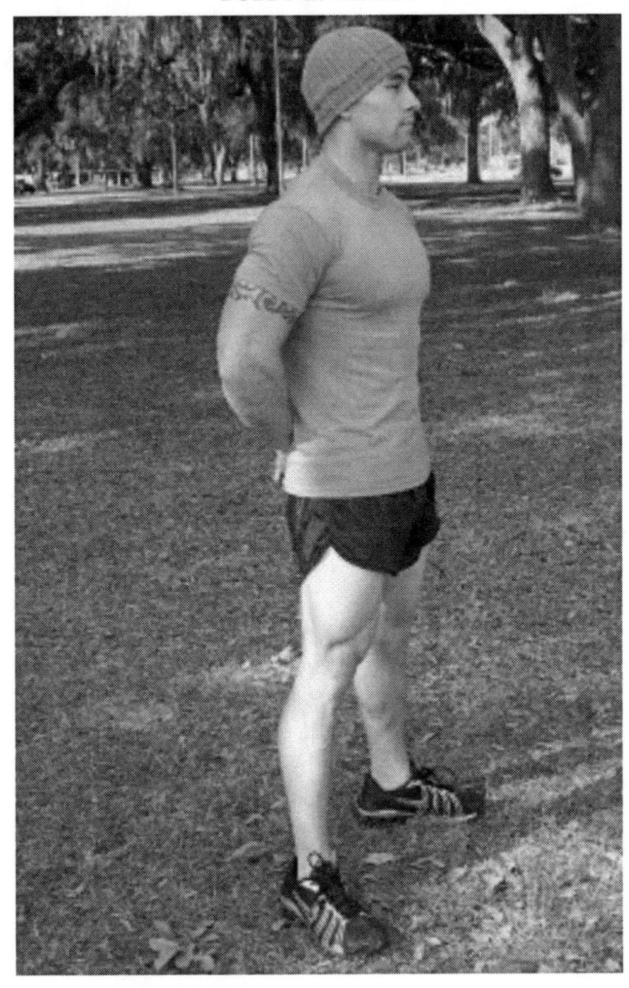

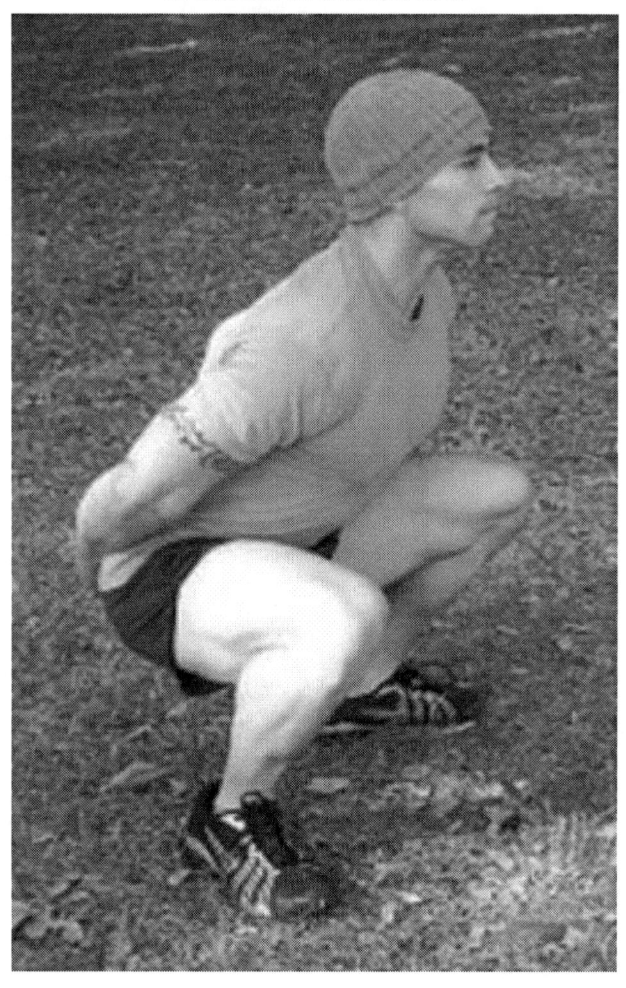

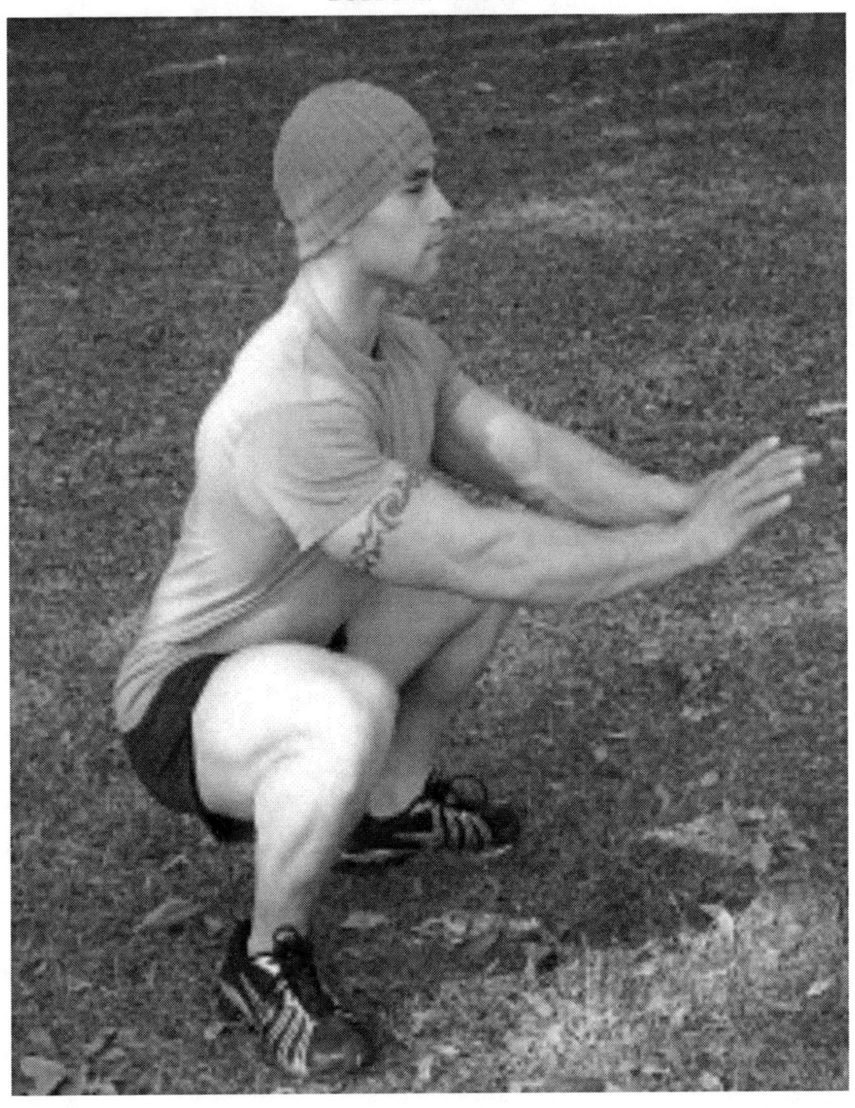

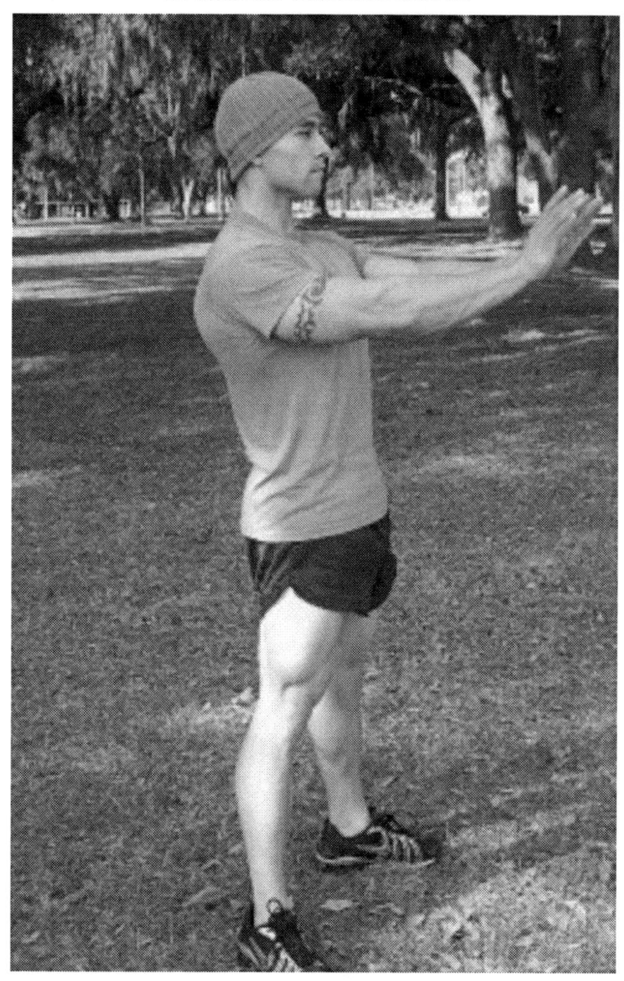

JUMP SQUATS: This exercise is great for developing your vertical jump and sprint speed.

<u>STEPS:</u>

1) Begin by standing with your feet shoulder-width apart and your hands resting at your sides.
2) Next squat down until your hands touch the ground.
3) Now explode up leaping as high in the air as you can. As you jump bring your arms up over your head then back down to your sides as you descend. Sounds simple doesn't it, well give them a try and see for yourself.

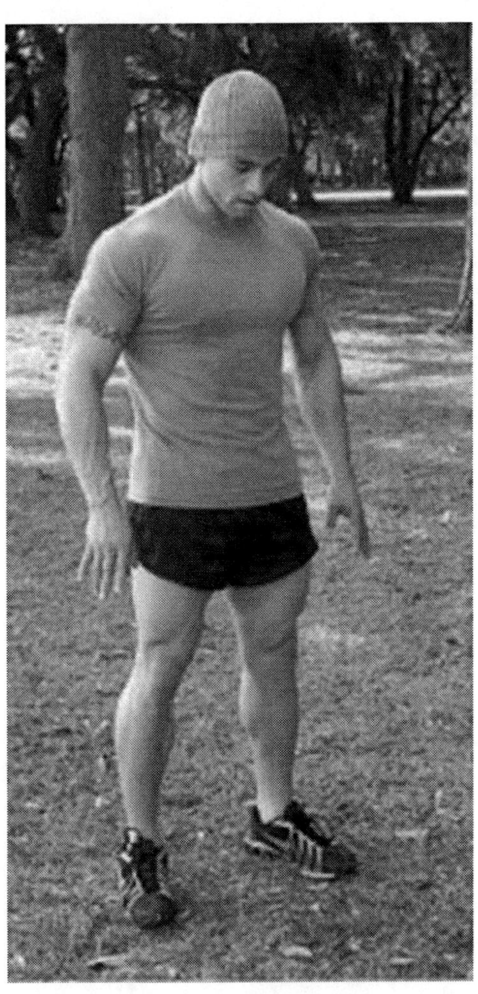

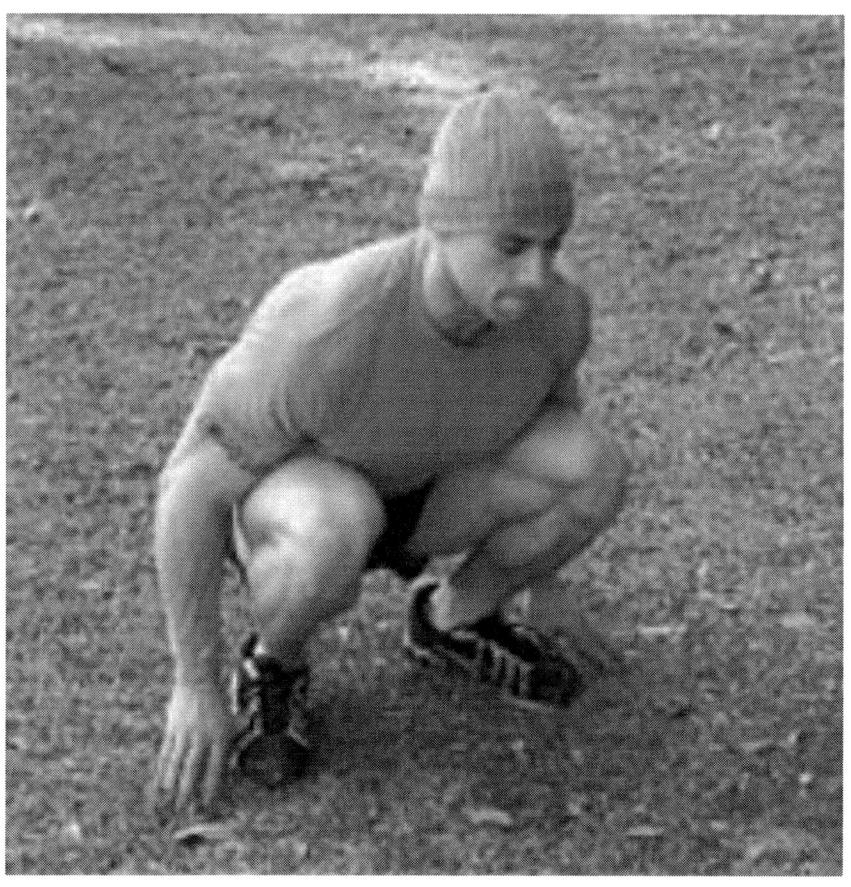

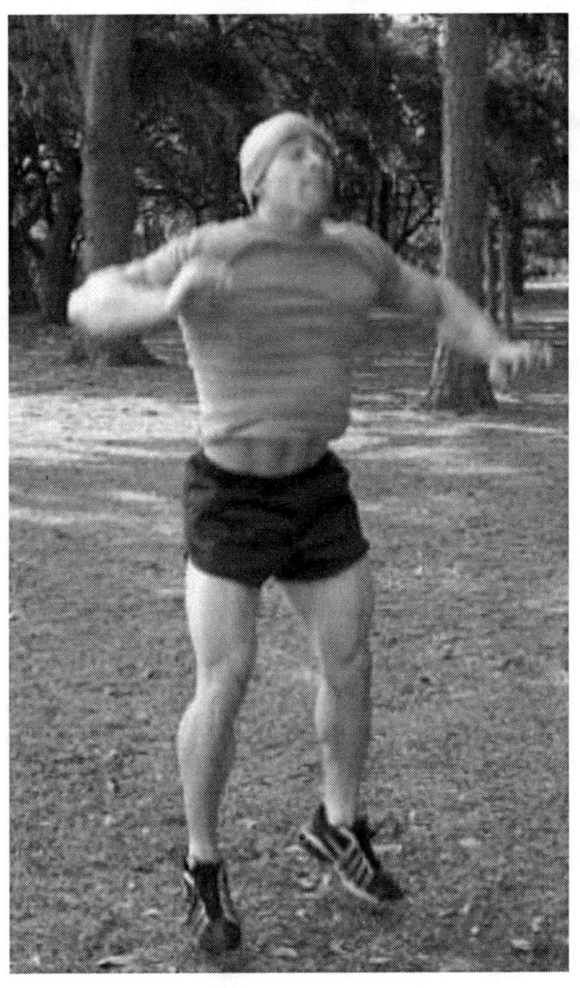

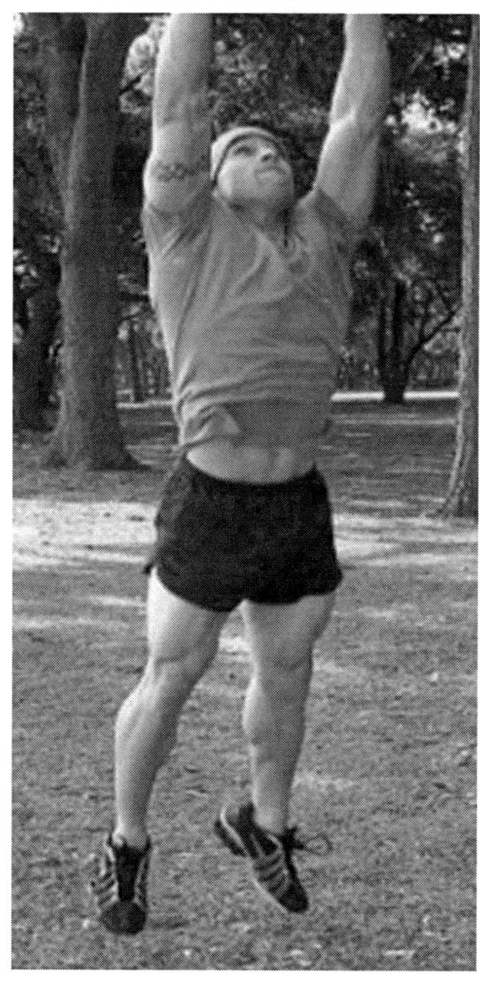

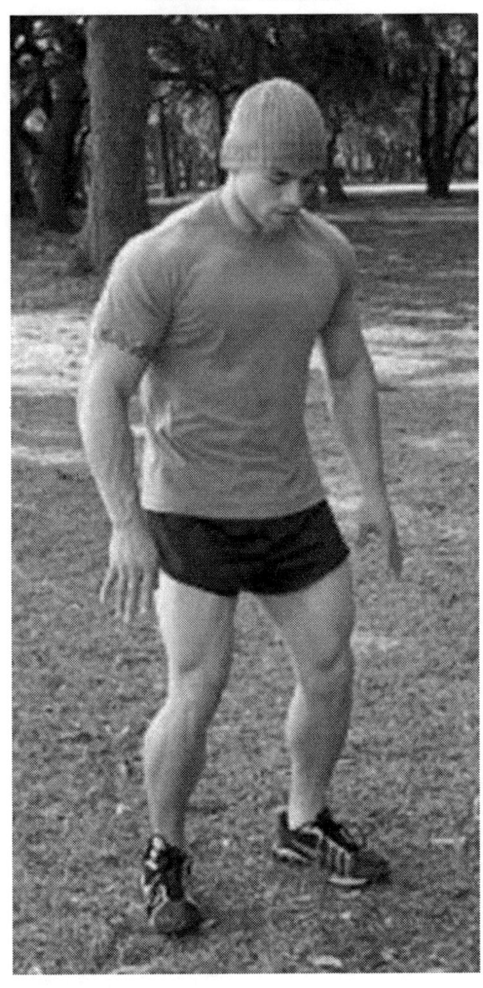

HILL SPRINTS AND HILL BOUNDS: Now the ultimate goal of this style of training is function. These two exercises are the epitome of functionalism by providing growth in speed, strength, agility, endurance, and muscularity. The important thing here is selecting a hill that is realistic to your capability. You should pick a hill that is approximately fifty to one hundred yards long. The slope of your hill will ultimately determine the length.

SPRINTS: Once you have selected your hill, the choices of routines are endless. But here are a few:

- 10 X 100 (10 sprints of 100 yards each)
- 100 pyramid (start with 100 yards, down to 50 increments of ten yards, then back up to 100)
- Backwards Sprints (Choose your distance, and sprint backwards for as many runs as desired).

BOUNDS: Here is the ultimate leg crippler. Once again, select a hill according to your capability.

STEPS:

1) Start at the bottom of your hill in a squatting position with your palms on the ground.
2) Now explode forward and up, jumping as high and far as you can. Then land back in the squat position.
3) You may see that it is necessary to utilize a small hop at the end of each jump to compensate for the extreme force and momentum.

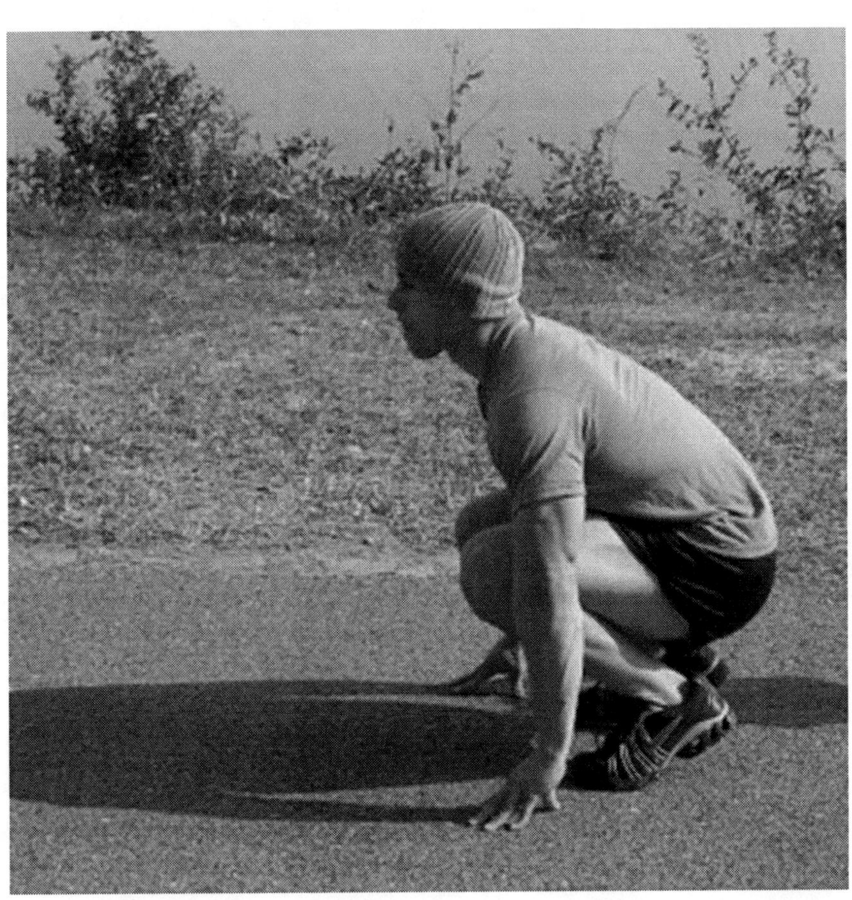

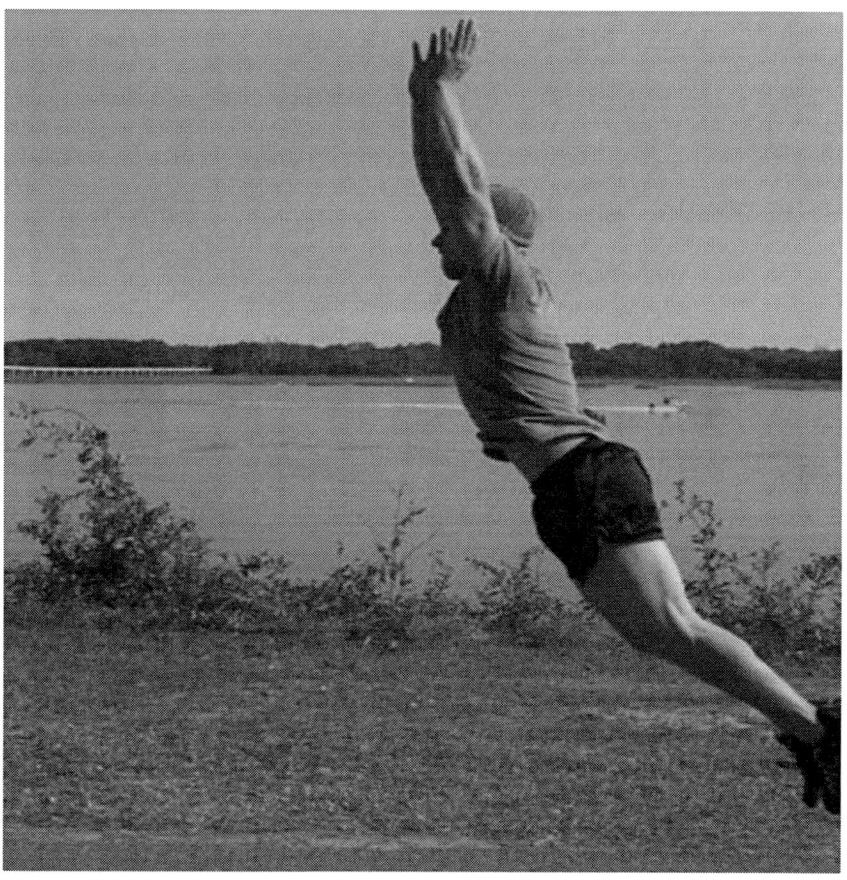

NOTE: Due to their extreme nature, ensure you warm up and stretch your entire body adequately before conducting any of these exercises.

CHAPTER 7

ABS:

"Train harder than you will ever have to perform."

LEG LIFTS: This exercise puts a lot of stress on the lower abdominals if done correctly.

STEPS:

1) Begin by lying on the floor in front of your couch or any other heavy object you can slip your fingers under. Your head should be at the couch with your body running perpendicular to the couch.
2) Slip your fingers under the bottom of the couch so that your hands are above your head.
3) From this position, simply raise your feet about six inches off the ground. This is your starting position.
4) From here you raise your legs up, creating a ninety-degree angle with your body.
5) Once you are at a ninety-degree, raise your hips off the ground as you complete your exhalation.
6) Now lower you hips. Then lower your legs back down ensuring your feet do not touch the ground. That was rep one.

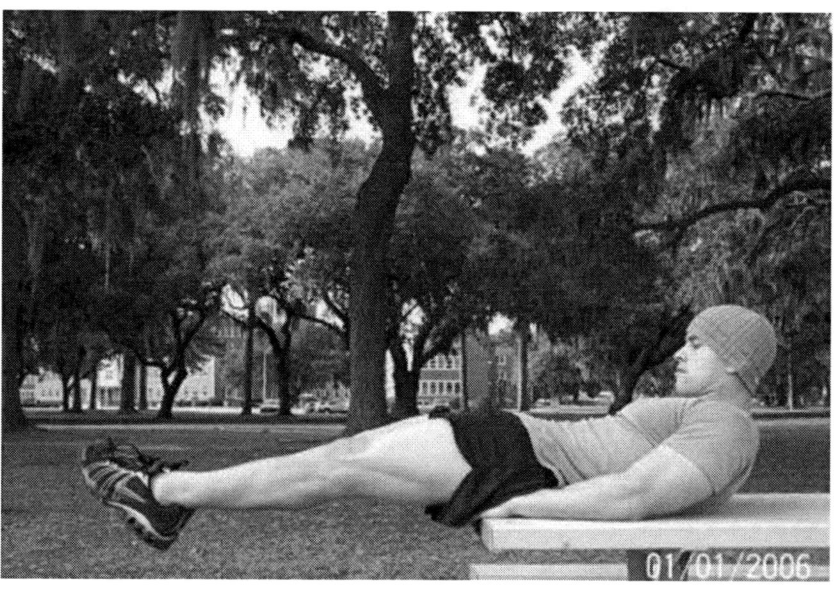

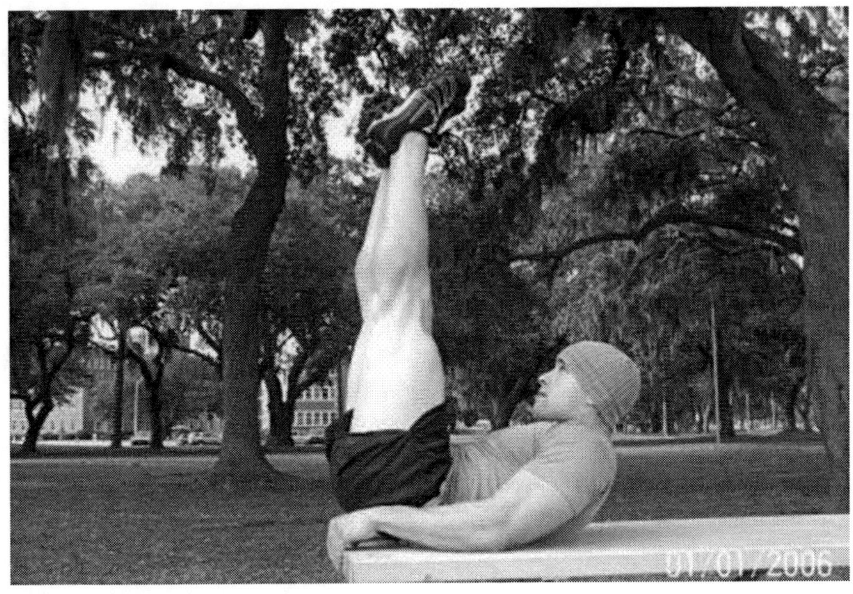
01/01/2006

SITOUTS: This exercise is based off a wrestling technique used to escape an opponent. It puts a lot of stress on your obliques if done correctly.

<u>**STEPS:**</u>

1) Starting position is exactly like that of the Hindu push-ups. Place palms on the ground, forming the inverted "V" with your body. Your feet are slightly more than shoulder width apart.
2) From here, take your right foot and shoot it underneath your body. Then attempt to place it just behind your left hand.
3) Now return your right foot back to its original position, simultaneously shooting your left foot to the right hand. This exercise takes some coordination and a little rhythm. Every time you kick a leg through, ensure you twist your hips.

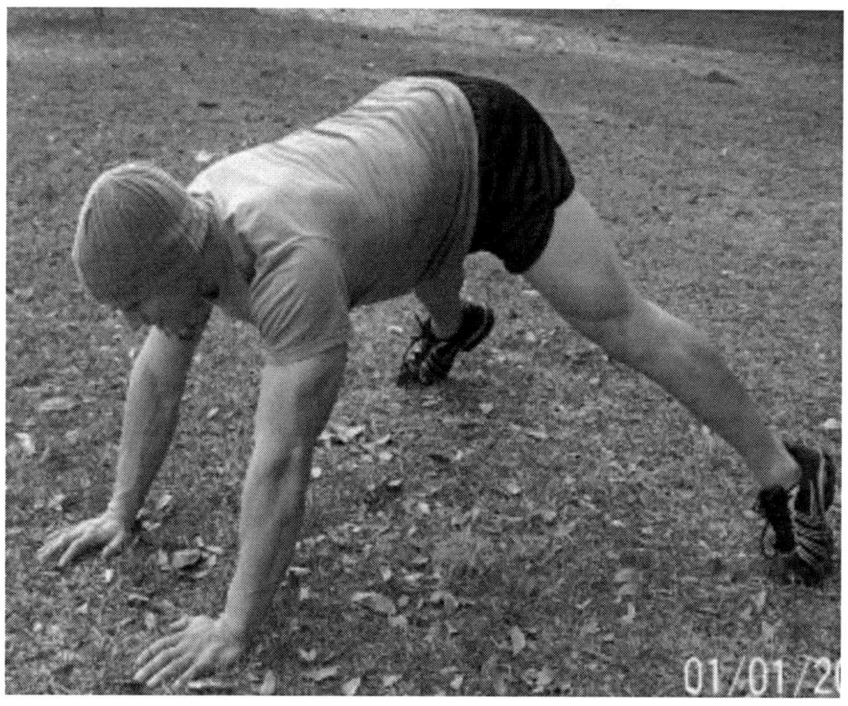

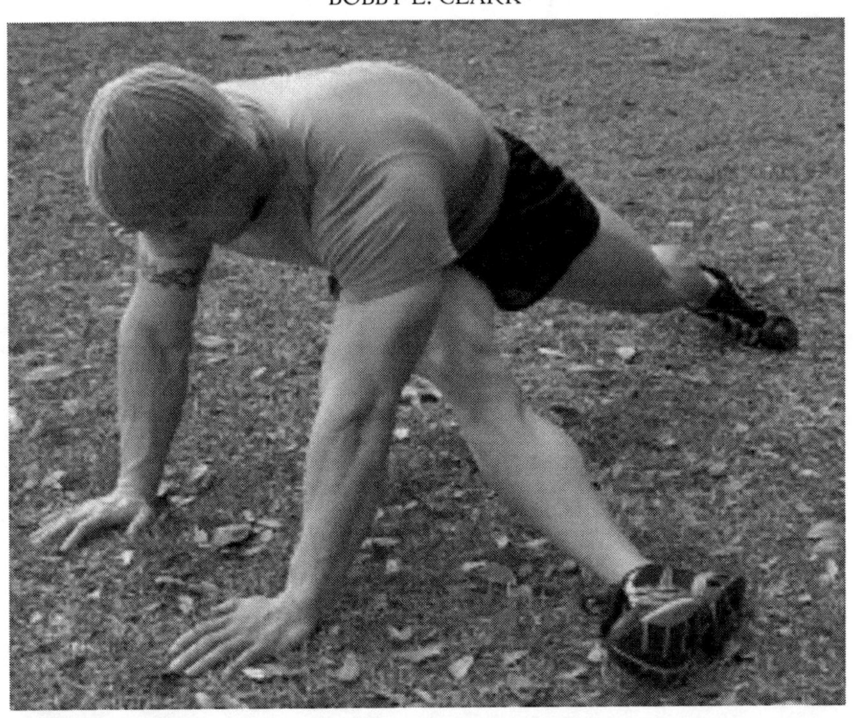

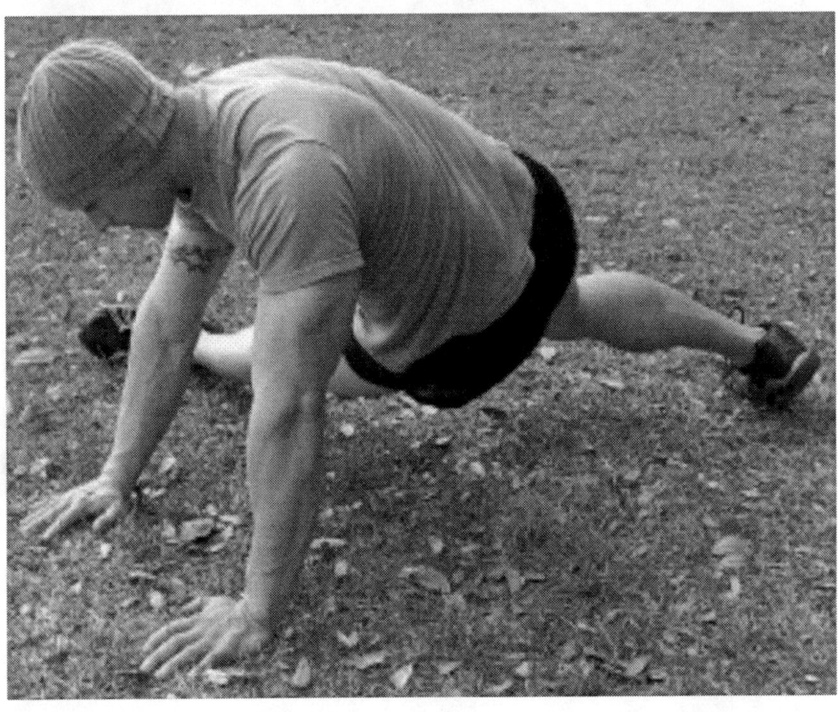

BICYCLES: This is the traditional exercise you probably are familiar with. It is awesome for the entire abdominal region—both front and sides.

STEPS:

I like to do this exercise on the edge of bench.

1) The starting position should be on your back with knee tucked to your chest, and the other leg is straight out, parallel with your body.
2) Your upper body should be crunched up with your hands placed at your ears, and your opposite elbow touching the knee that is up.
3) From here simply alternate your legs simultaneously with the opposite elbow. Your leg that is extended should be straight out, stretching your abdominals and hip flexor. All the work should be done with your abs.

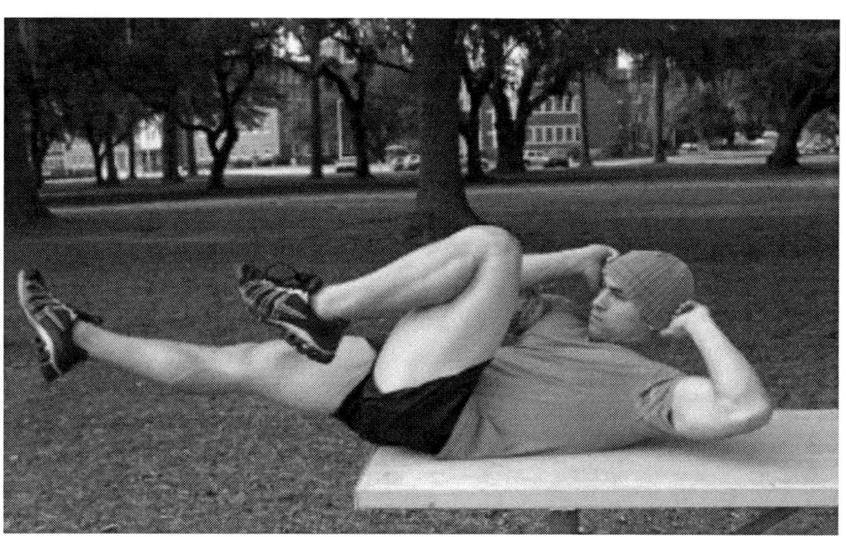

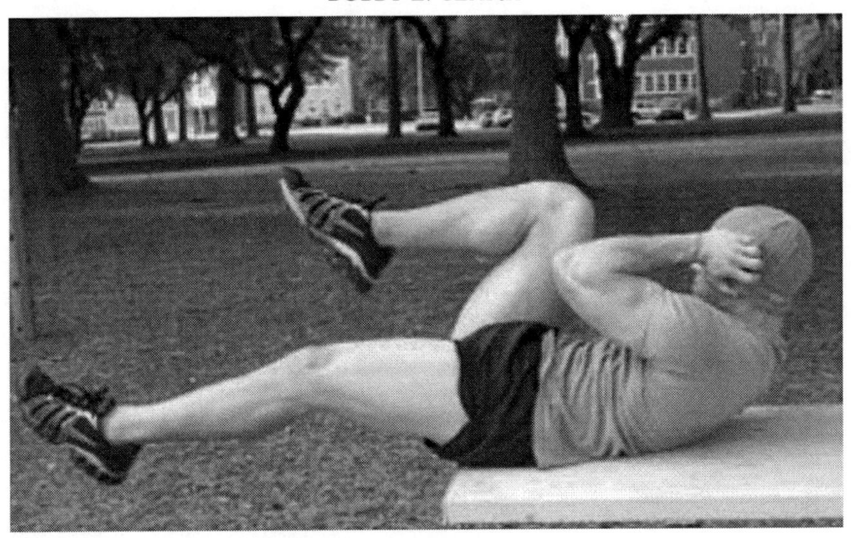

"V" UPS: These are an awesome exercise for the entire front abdominal wall.

<u>**STEPS:**</u>

1) Begin on your back with your hands together, reaching out above your head.
2) Begin the movement by raising your feet and hands simultaneously attempting to touch your toes with your hands. Don't jerk or use momentum.
3) As you come back down from the up position, control your descent all the way down. Do not let your feet hit the ground. Stop them at about six inches from the ground. That's one rep.

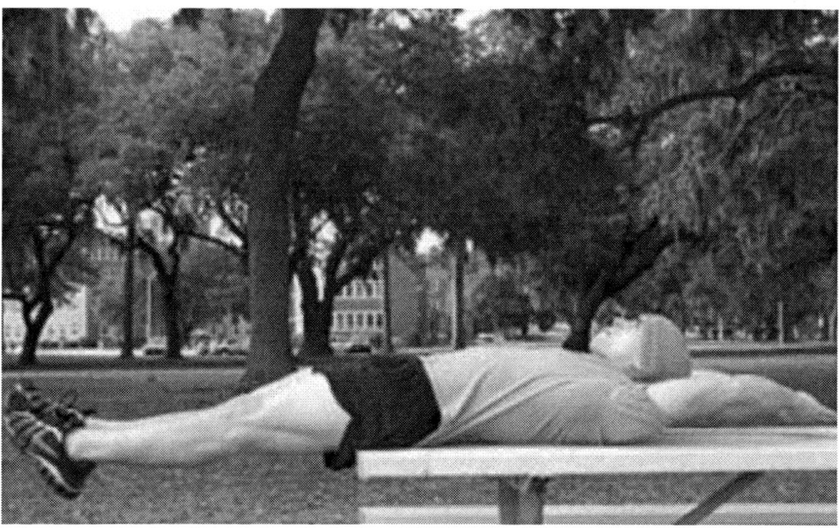

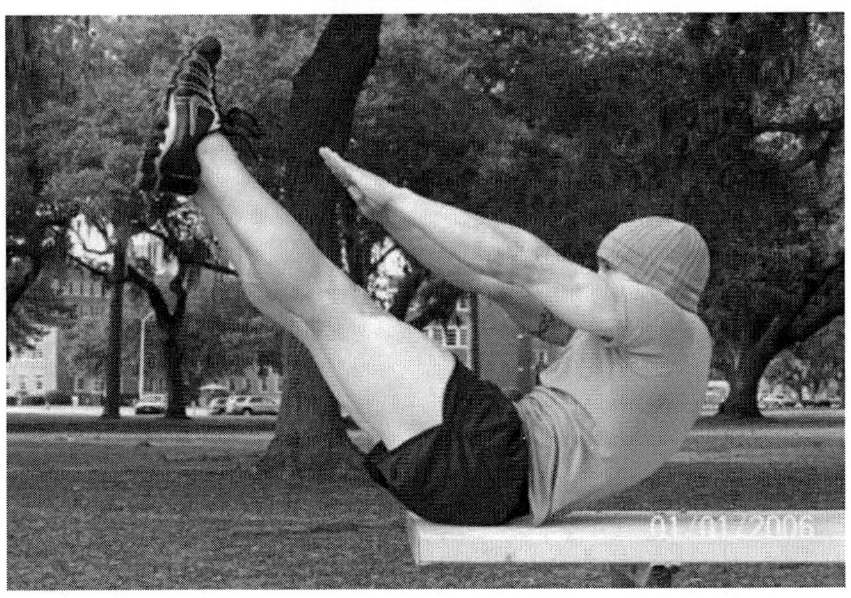
01/01/2006

"180/45/90s": This exercise is all about isolation. This is one exercise I use mainly in my circuit courses.

STEPS:

1) These exercises are best accomplished by using a bench. You need to be elevated so that your legs can hang further than 180 degrees when laying flat on the end of the bench.
2) From this position, raise you straight legs up to about a forty-five-degree angle and hold for a predetermined count.
3) Once you reach your count, raise you legs up to ninety degrees. So now your body should be in an "L" shape with your legs in the air.
4) Once you've reached your count at ninety degrees, bring your legs back down to forty-five degrees, hold, then back down to 180 and hold. Continue through the repetitions until you've reached your overall set time limit for your circuit.

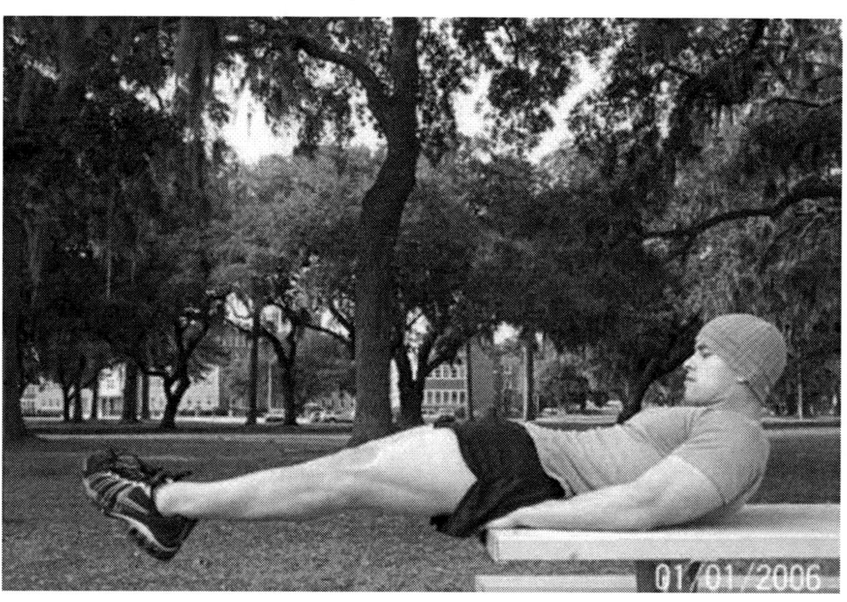

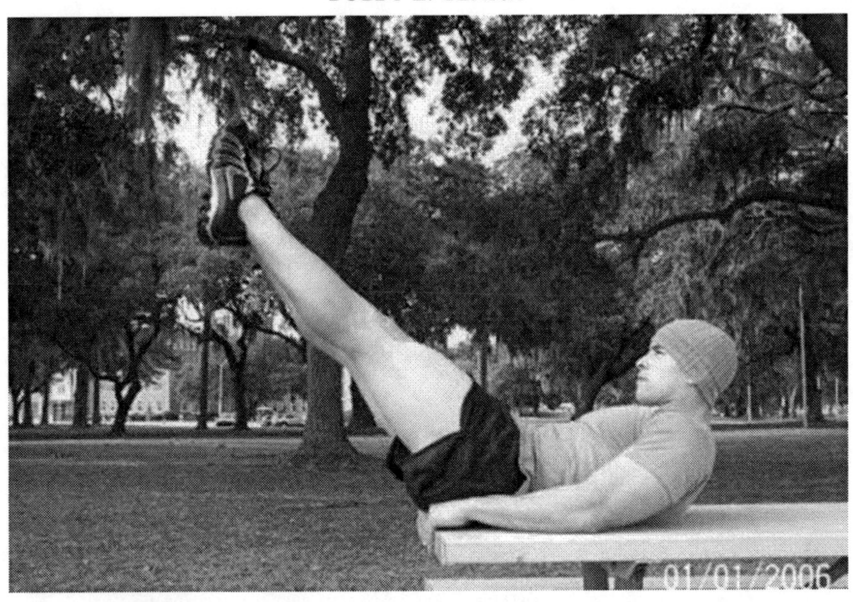
01/01/2006

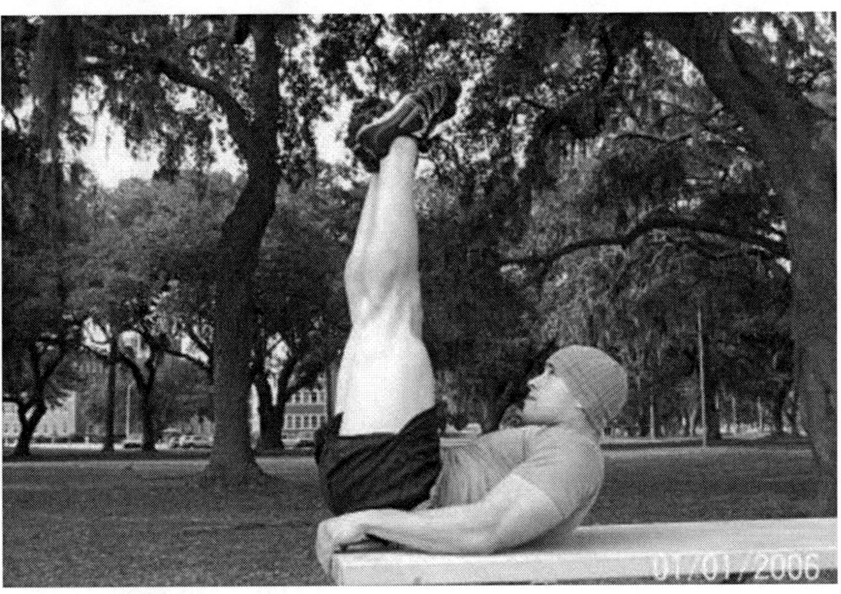
01/01/2006

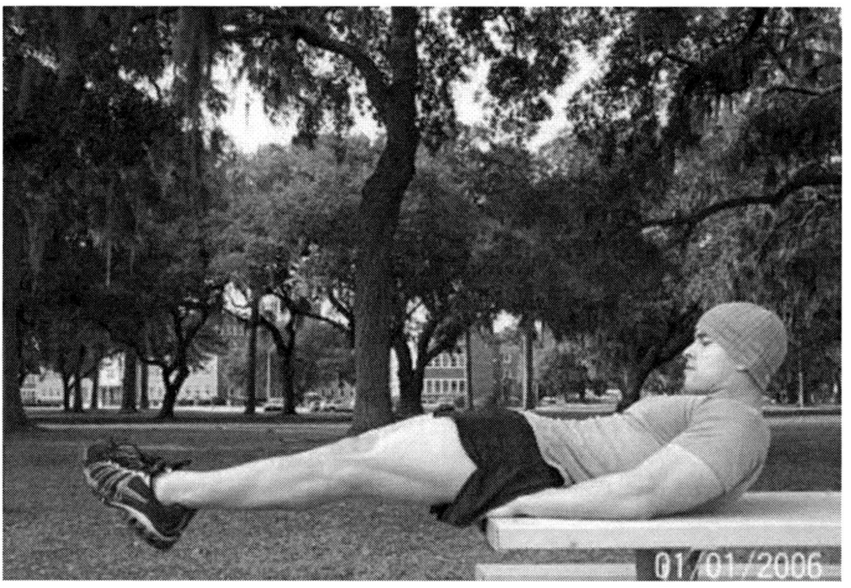
01/01/2006

CHAPTER 8

ROAD WORK

"You are in complete control of your legacy. How do you want to be remembered?"

Running is one of those exercises that I find to be extremely beneficial and a must in any exercise program. I have found that most people just flat out don't enjoy running. Then again, most people don't enjoy working out either. First, I also noticed that the majority of the individuals who don't enjoy running don't understandhow to run correctly. And secondly, they believe running is simply getting from Point "A" to Point "B" as fast as they can. When in actuality, running has just as many variations as ice cream has flavors. I have included in this section a breakdown of my running techniques as well as a handful of running exercises.

TECHNIQUE:

Running is simply using gravity to pull you down the road. Here is how it is done. When you run, try and lean forward—almost to the point that you have to move your legs to stay up. As you trot down the road stay on the balls of your feet and try and pull each step rather than push. You'll notice that if you pull your feet to your butt you will utilize your hamstring more than your quads and place less impact on your knees. By running with a pull in your step rather than a push, you are also minimizing the resistance your feet create at each impact they have with the ground. Finally stay light on your feet and keep your body relaxed. This will ensure the energy you use isn't wasted on useless exertion. It may take a while for you to grasp this technique, but once you do—you'll reap the benefits.

RUNNING OPTIONS:

INTERVAL RUNNING: This is a timed interval so you'll need a watch. Start out at a normal pace until you are good and warm. Now set your timer for thirty seconds. When you are ready, sprint for thirty seconds. Once your watch beeps, slow back down to your original pace. Run at this pace now for two minutes then back to the thirty-second sprint. You can create you own intervals with backwards sprints, bounds, lunges, etc. Your imagination is the limit.

PUSH AND RUN: This run is a killer for both your upper and lower body. Take off on your run at whatever distance you want. I suggest at least three miles. Once you are warmed up, stop and do twenty, four-count push-ups (starting position is up, go down for a count of one, back up for a count of two, back down for a count of three, and back up for a four count). Get up and continue running with no rest between pushing and running. After you've continued running for about a quarter mile, stop again. Now you are doing twenty Hindu push-ups. Get back up and continue running. Keep up with the quarter-mile, running and alternating between push-ups and Hindu push-ups. You can utilize any exercises you want to make endless varieties of this run.

WEIGHT RUN: Not too difficult to figure this one out. Grab two dumbbells (I use ten pound weights). Get on the road and run. If you get tired hold the weight up on your shoulders, but don't put them down. This run will really take it out of you, especially if you don't cheat.

THE MACHINE'S TOOL BOX

A COLLECTION OF MY FAVORITE WORKOUTS

CIRCUIT TRAINING

Initially, let us talk a little about circuit training. This method of training is awesome for developing unparalleled muscular endurance and stamina—not to mention a mean pump that'll shred the body. There are two ways to go about conducting circuit training: Timed and Repetition. Timed training is simply determining the amount of time you will conduct a technique. For instance, one minute of continuous exercise. Then you determine the amount of time you will rest—thirty seconds. After your thirty-second rest, conduct another minute of your timed exercise. Repetition circuit training is simple as well. First determine the amount of repetitions you will accomplish. Once you accomplish that determined amount, rest for a second or two. Then move on to the next exercise. Adding addition reps ever other week or so develops this type of circuit training, depending on your ability. Now that you have a grasp on the two types of circuit training, whip it on!

CIRCUIT WORKOUTS:

- Hindu squats
- Ballistic push-ups
- Chest pull-ups
- Jump squats
- Hindu push-ups
- Fifteens

CIRCUIT TWO:

- Ballistic push-ups
- Lunges
- Sit-outs
- Hindu push-ups
- Mountain Climbers
- 180/45/90s

CIRCUIT THREE:

- Alternating push-ups
- Hindu Squats
- Bicycles
- Perpendicular push-ups
- One-legged wall sits
- Leg lifts

CIRCUIT FOUR:

- Press-ups
- Jump Squats
- V-ups
- Push-ups
- Mountain Climbers
- Inverted Leg lifts

EIGHT COUNT BODY BUILDER

These little guys are a treat for your stamina, circulation, strength, and muscular endurance. They go great in circuit course or by them selves. Though there are many different variations, the method I'm going to explain to you is the one that I found emphasizes strength and stamina the best.

- Start with your feet about shoulder width apart, with your hands to your side.
- Keeping your feet flat on the ground and your back straight, lower your body until you can place your palms flat on the ground in front of you. *Count one.*
- Now kick your feet straight back so you are in the "up" position of a push-up, *Count two.*
- From this position you conduct two controlled push-ups. *Down three, up four, down five, up six.*
- Now bring your feet back under you until they are once again flat on the ground: *Count seven.*
- The last step in the movement is to stand back up. Do it controlled while pushing from your heals. It should not be fast, instead it should be with emphasis on control: *Count eight.*

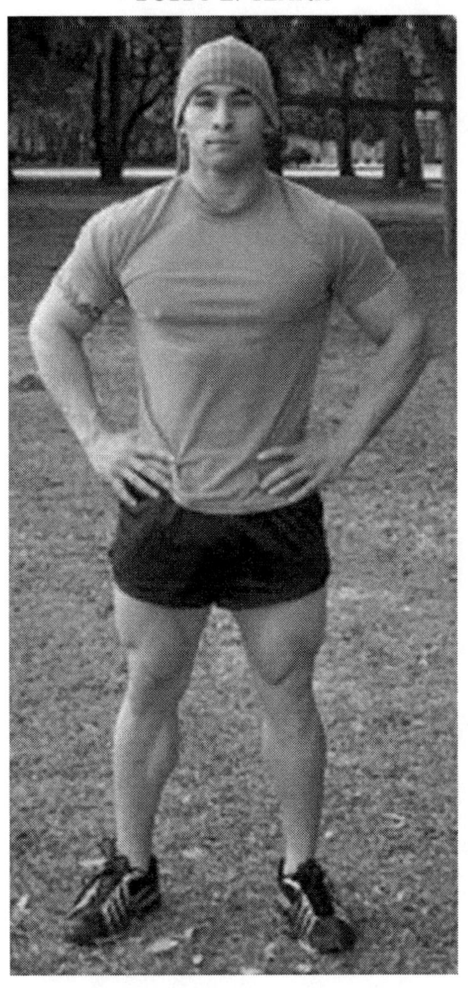

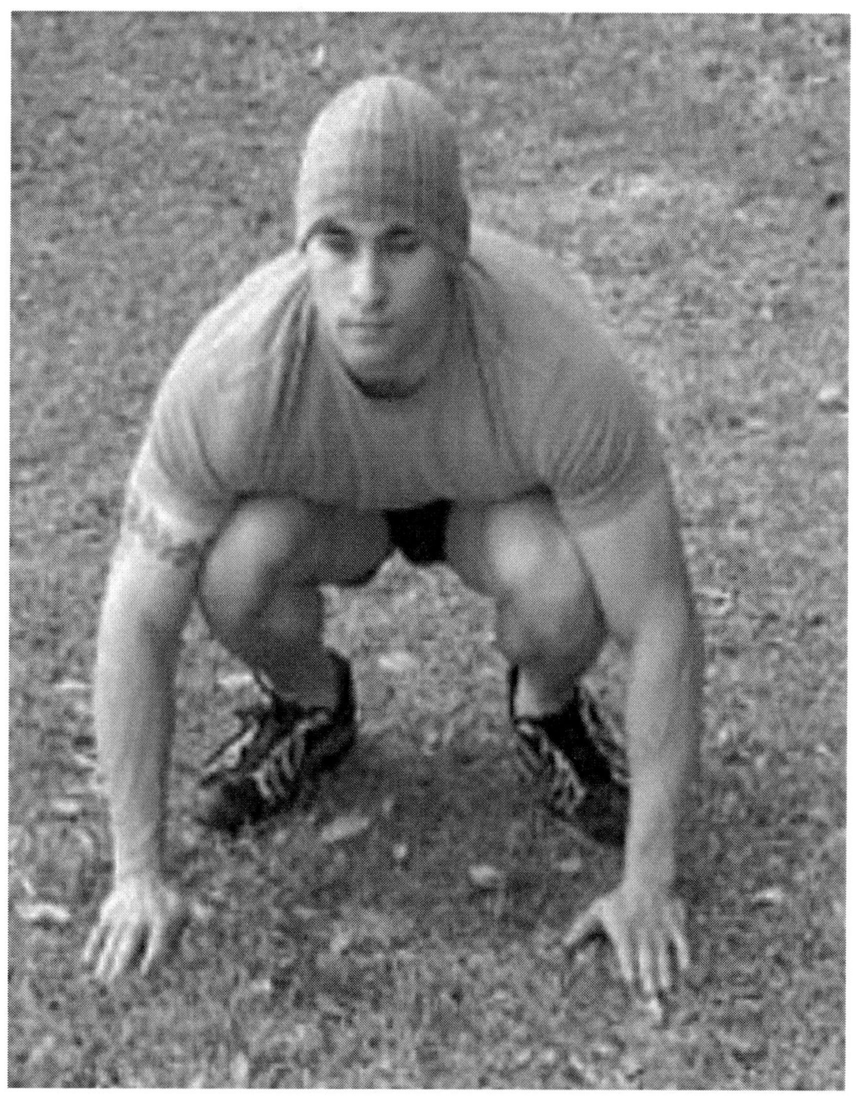

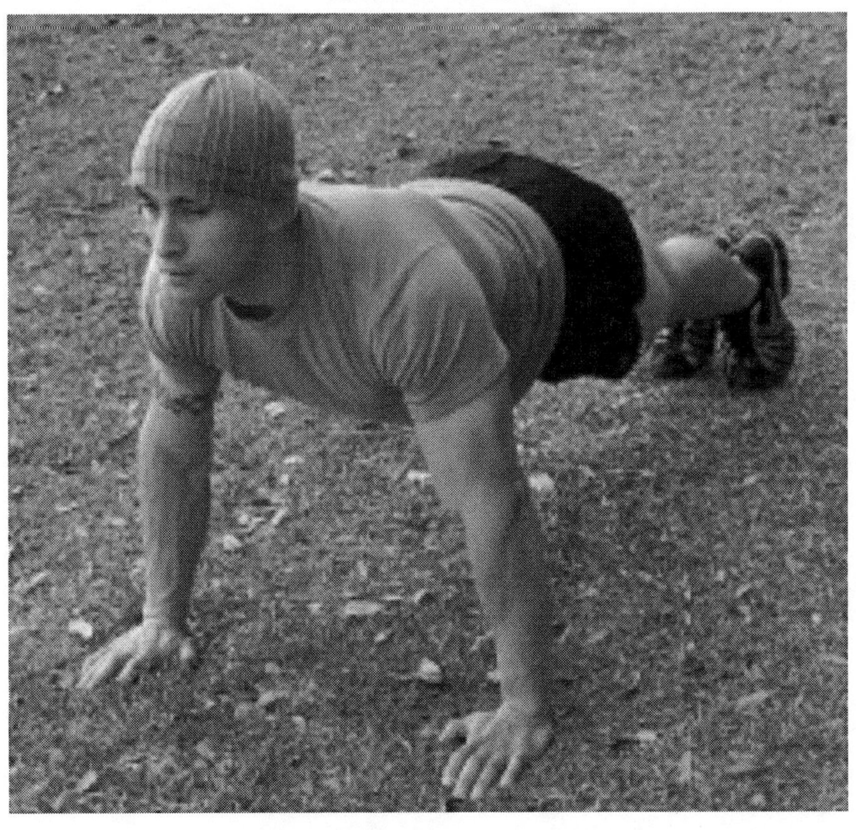

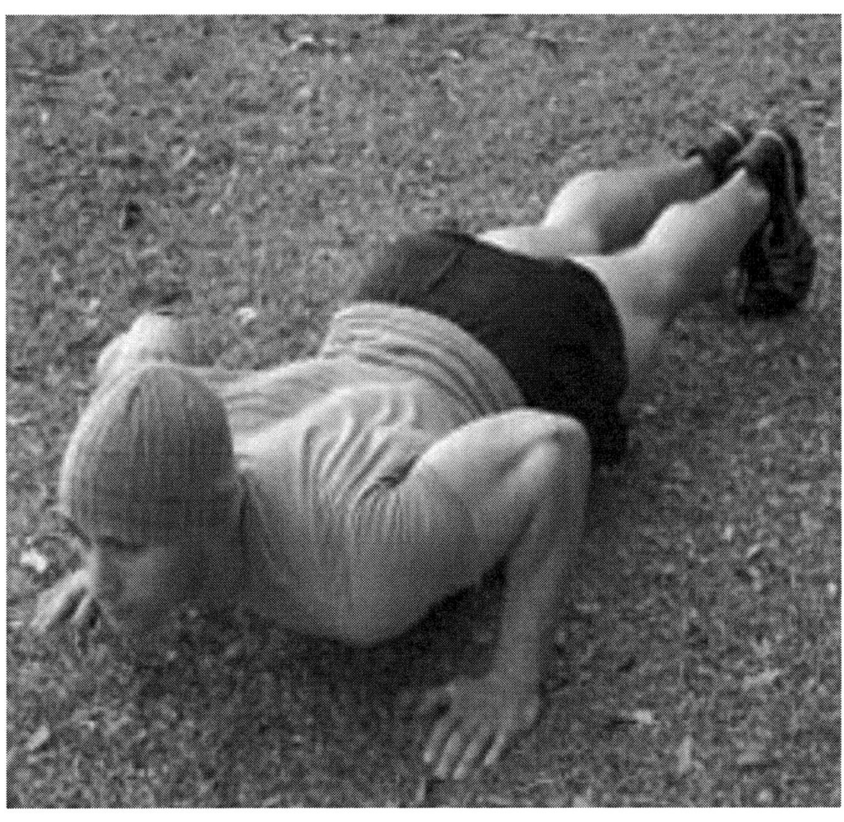

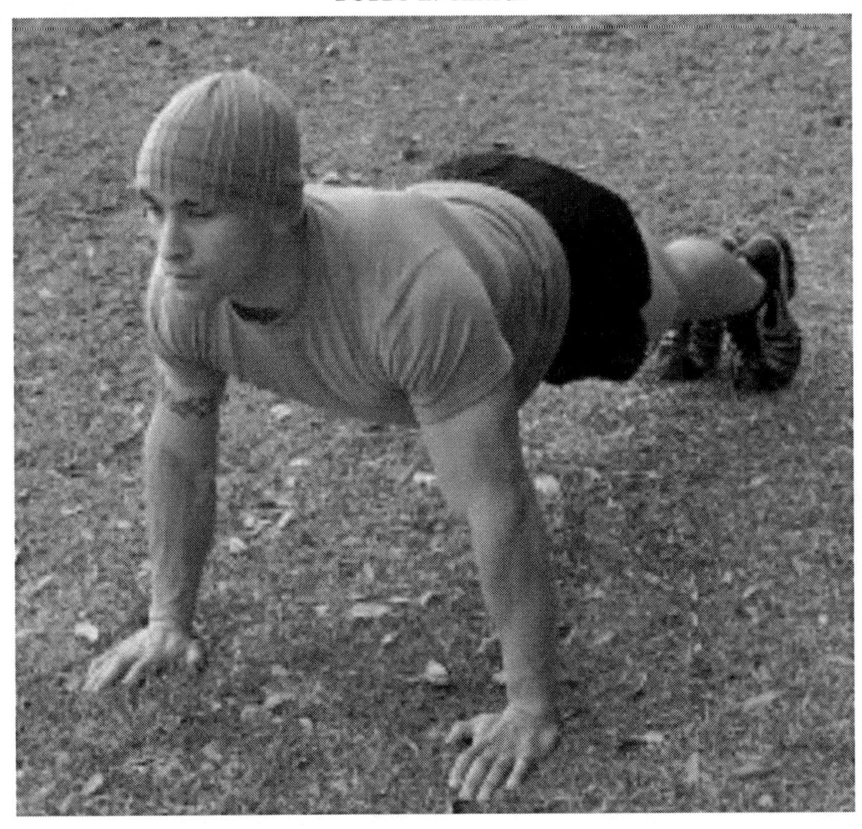

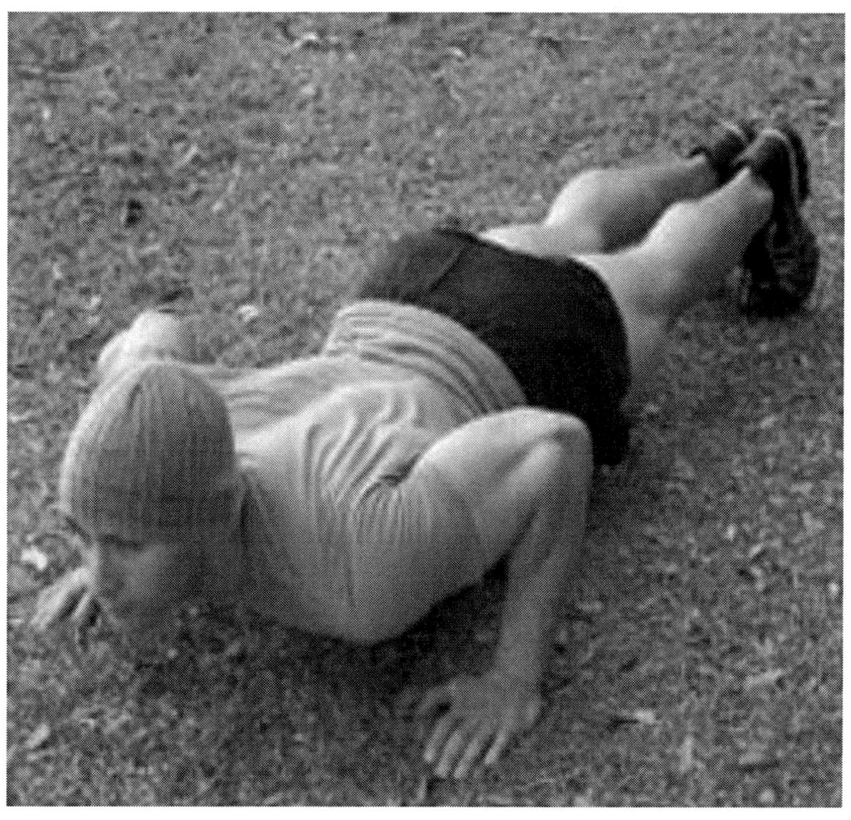

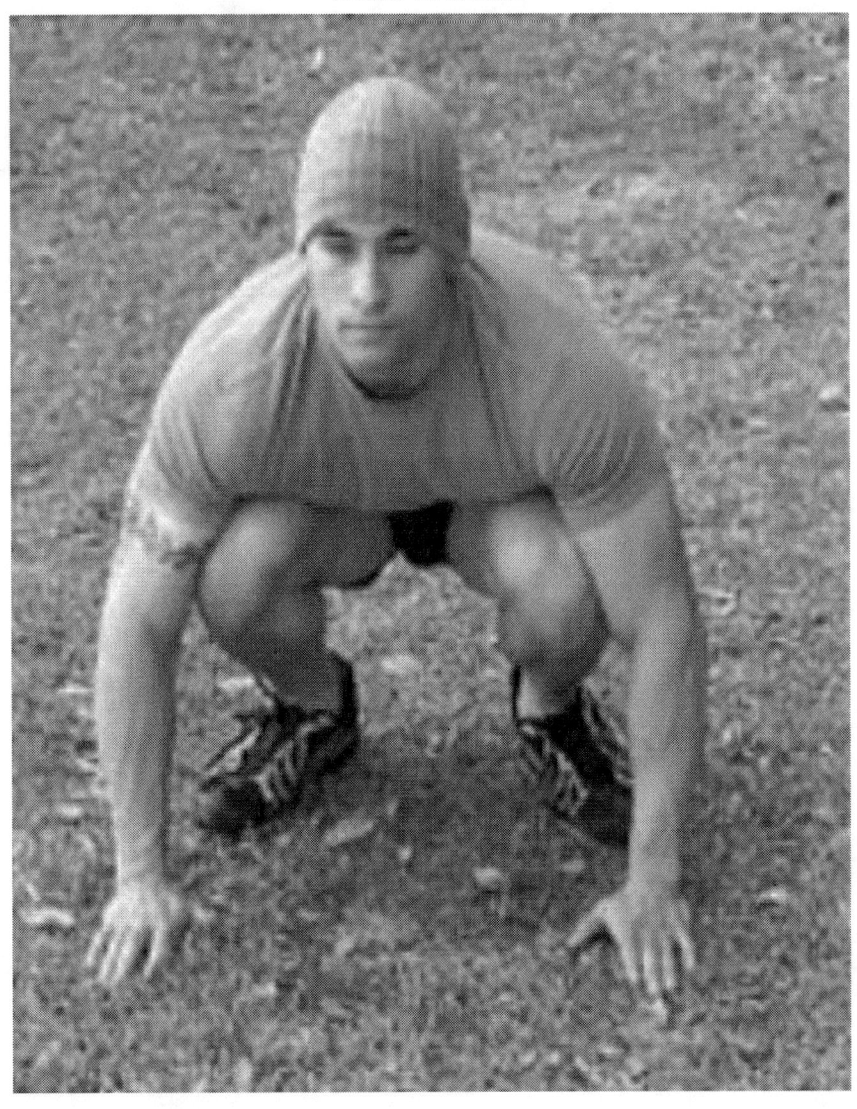

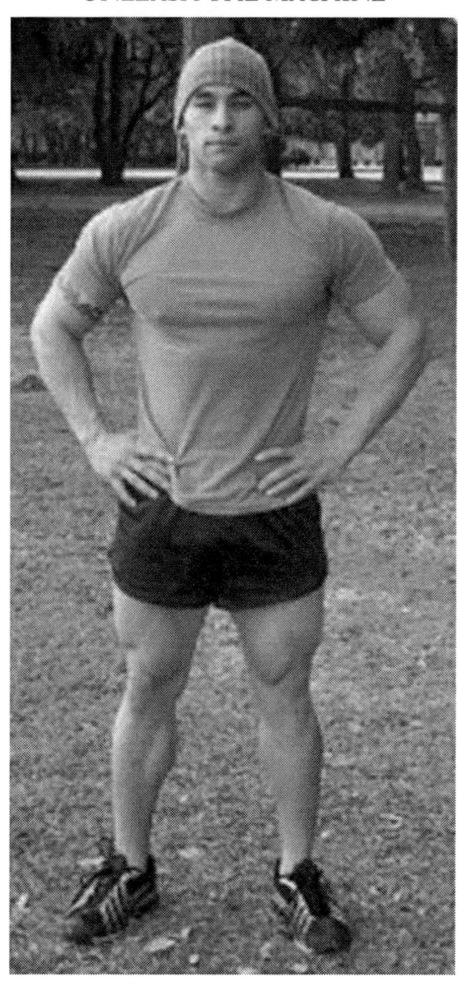

WORKOUTS WITH THE BODY BUILDER

WORKOUT ONE:

I have two main workouts that I do with the eight counts. The first is simple sets of fifty. Start with fifty and work your way down to zero non-stop. Now you may have to adjust the count, but the goal is to get at least four sets with no more than one minute rest between each set. You will see that this workout is a great way to kill your body.

WORKOUT TWO:

The second workout is a combination of the eight counts and mountain climbers. Depending on your condition, you may want to start with about twenty to twenty-five reps. And once again the goal is four sets with no more that one minute rest between each set. The exercise is simple. You just alternate from body builders to the mountain climbers, then rest. You will soon see that this exercise hurts (in a good way of course).

PRISON YARD WORKOUT

300 X 5:

This little workout isn't for the average person. It consists of one exercise—pull-ups. Utilizing both variations of grip, the goal is exactly as it sounds, 300 pull-ups in one hour by doing five repetitions every minute. It's a great way to spend an hour and break down your back and arms.

300 X 5 X 2:

This is a variation of the previous workout, *with a twist.* The same principals apply—five pull-ups every minute. The change is an addition of five dips per minute. Initially you will probably want to start with a thirty-minute workout and gradually work your way to one hour. This exercise hurts, so you want to make sure you are adequately warmed up.

WEIGHTED WORKOUT:

This routine involves three different exercises with a buddy. The three different exercises are pull-ups, dips, and buddy push-ups. You will need a chain belt, weights, a pull-up bar, and dip bars. Begin with one of the three exercises. (I usually start with dips.) Complete four sets of four to six reps. You need to adjust your weight to enable you to only get that number of reps. After you and your partner complete all four sets of dips, move the pull-up bar. Once again adjust the weight allowing you to get four to six reps. Finally move to the push-ups. Have your partner apply just enough pressure to allow only four to six reps. This exercise is a mass building exercise, and it must be conducted with perfect form for best results.

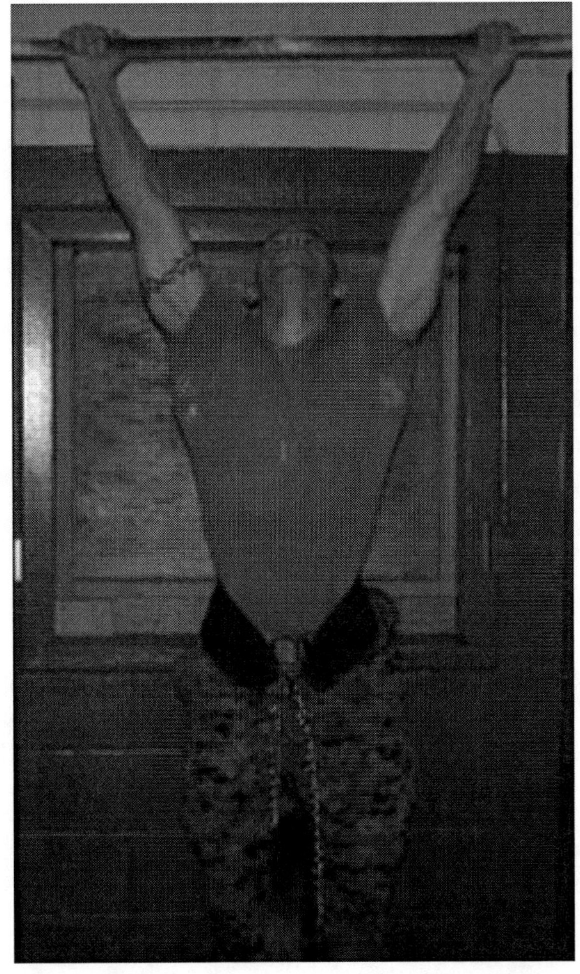

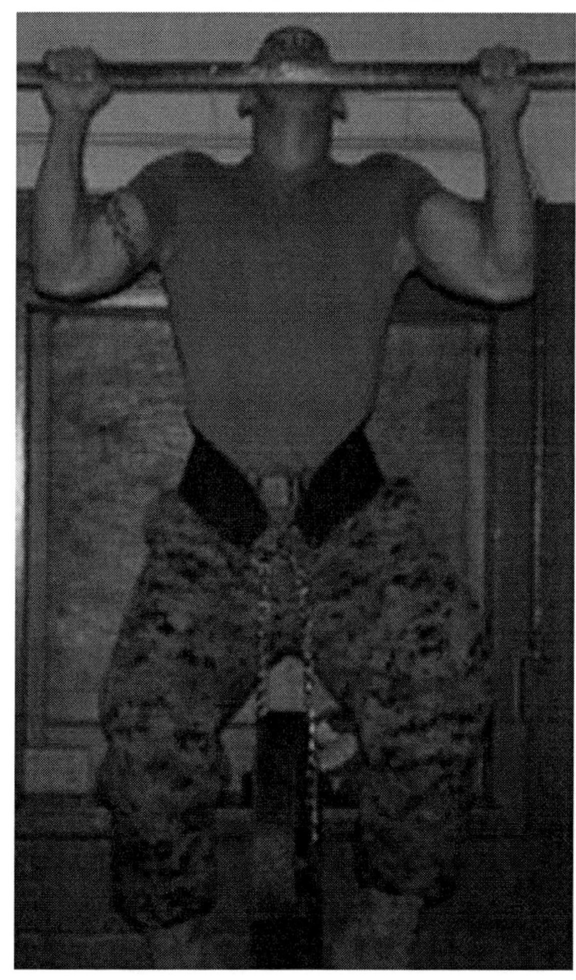

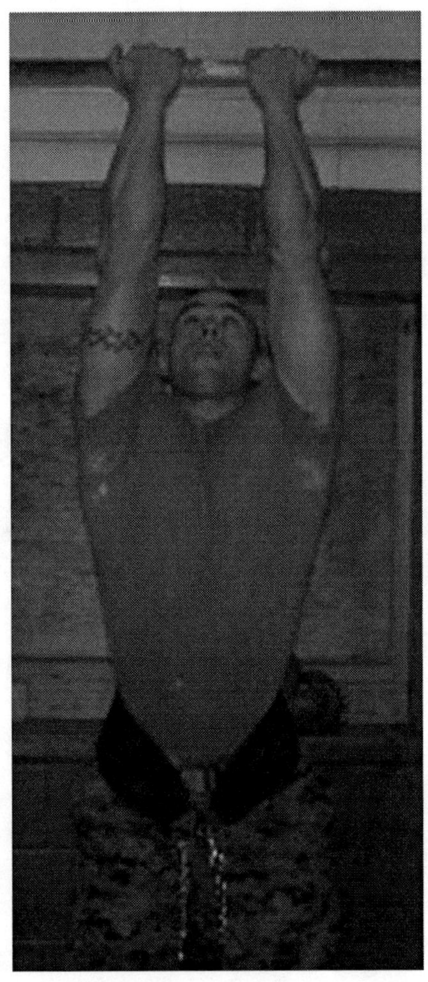

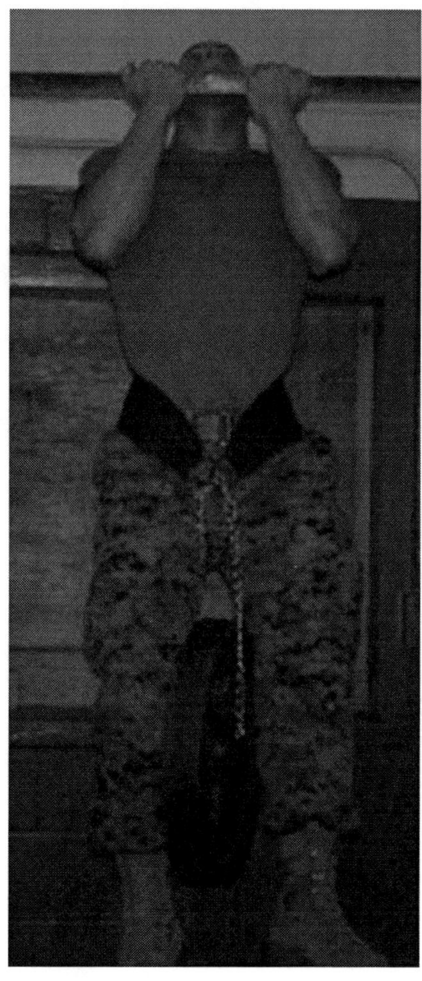

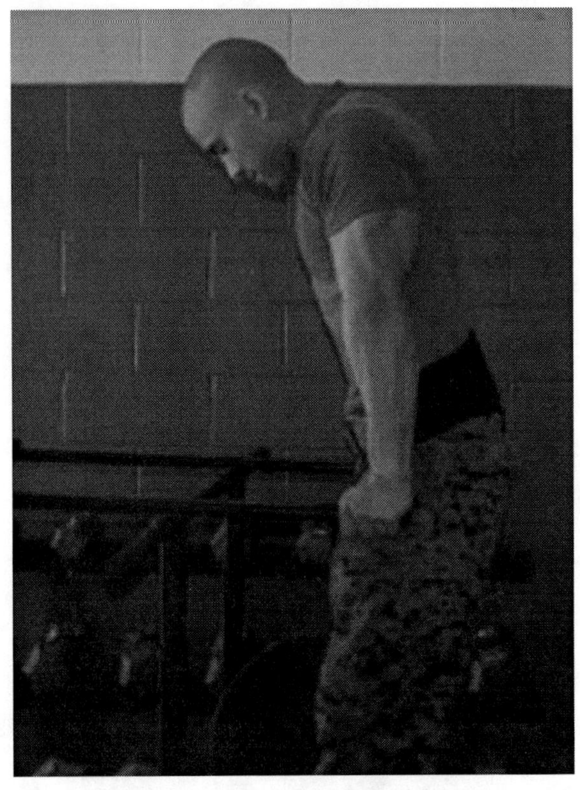

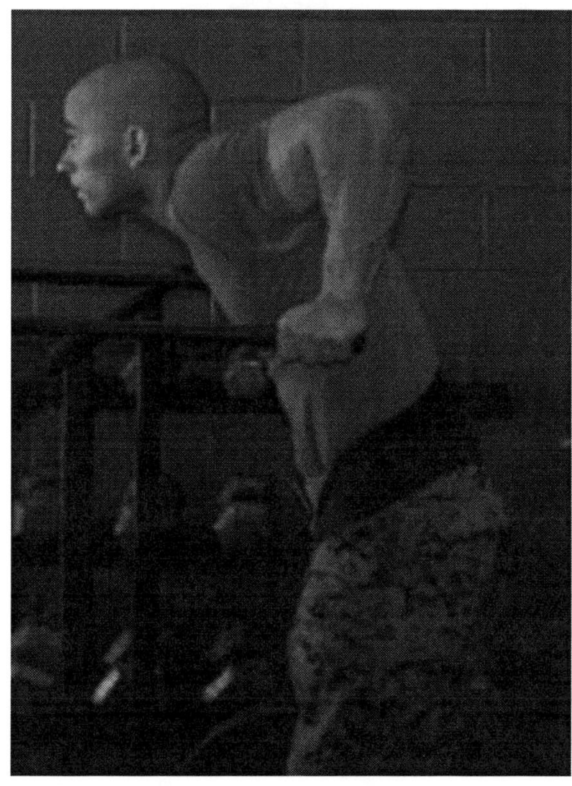

THE MACHINE'S WEEK LONG PLAN:

This is a weeklong plan I put together basically as a format that you can modify to fit your fitness level.

DAY 1—DAY 5-

SHOULDERS:
Handstand push-ups-**4 x Max**
1-3-5 Handstand push-ups-**4 x Max**
Hindu push-ups-**4 x Max**
BI'S:
ISO Pull-ups-**4 x Max**
1-3-5 ISO Pull-ups-**4 x Max**
15's-**4 sets**
One arm pull-ups-**4 x Max**
ABS:
Leg lifts-**Max reps +10**
Sit outs-**Max reps**
Bicycles-**Max reps +10**

DAY 2—DAY 6-

TRI'S:
One arm push-ups-**4 x Max**
1-3-5 Diamond push-ups-**4 x Max**
Hammer push-ups-**4 x Max**
High and Tights-**4 x Max**
BACK:
Gorillas-**4 x Max**
1-3-5 pull-ups-**4 x Max**
Chest pull-ups-**4 x Max**
Leg bends-**4 x Max**

DAY 3—DAY 7-

CHEST:

Buddy push-ups-**4 x Max**
Ballistic push-ups-**4 x Max**
Alternating push-ups-**4 x Max**
Perpendicular Push-ups-**3 x 1 min**
LEGS:
One-legged Squats-**4 x Max**
Hindu Squats-**4 x 50**
Jump squats-**4 x 20**
Hill sprints-**10 x 100 yds**
Hill Bounds-**5 x 50 yds**
ABS:
Leg lifts-**Max reps +10**
Sit outs-**Max reps**
Bicycles-**Max reps +10**

DAY 4-

REST

CARD P.T. (PHYSICAL TORTURE)

If you are one of those people who are always on the go, this workout is tailor-made for you. It's real simple. All you need is a deck of ordinary playing cards. I like to call it my travel gym. Ok, this is how to do it you select two exercises. I have provided you with my choices in order of difficulty, easiest to most difficult. Next you decide which exercise will be the red cards and which will be the black. Shuffle your deck and begin, each card you flip will be the face value in repetitions. Face cards are ten, and aces are eleven. The Jokers are another set of the previous flipped card. Sounds fun doesn't it? Here is my break down of exercises by difficulty level:

Hindu push-ups/Hindu squats
Lunges/Ballistic push-ups
Mountain climbers/Eight count body builders
Jump Squats/Pull-ups
Perpendicular push-ups/Chest pull-ups
One-legged squats/Gorillas

IN CONCLUSION...

Developing and writing this book has been difficult at times but an extremely exciting adventure. From the moment I decided to write down my training routines, to perfecting the exercises and translating them into a written manual, I knew I was embarking on a revolutionizing project. Even with all the work and modifications I poured into this book, it is not a complete package.

Please understand that this book is not the only tool you need to develop your mind and body into my so-called "MACHINE." Though the book provides challenging and result-driven exercises, there are also other ingredients required to build and maintain the desired higher levels of fitness.

Aside from the training aspect of fitness, the second necessity is diet. You MUST create a diet plan that promotes muscular growth and fat loss that is tailored for your body and metabolism. There are many sources currently published which provide you a good foundation to build upon. But after all is said and done, every diet takes some level of customizing to satisfy each individual. The key to success isn't in finding a diet that works, but making a diet that works.

This is two of the three key elements in transforming your body from what it is now into a "MACHINE." The third key element is often neglected or overlooked as a necessity. Mental focus; conquering your mind is and will always be the most difficult challenge you will have to endure. Throughout my life my number one adversary has always been my own mind. For you it is no different. Now this powerful aspect of training is actually two-fold. The first part has to do with **focus and maintaining concentration** not only through out a workout, but throughout your life. It is detrimental that you train your mind to operate as proficient and focused as possible. No matter what time of day it is or what distractions occur, you must maintain. I call this mental stamina. The second part of the mental factor is **self-doubt**. That simple thought that invades your mind when you're tired, and when you feel weak. That voice that says "No more, just stop, and I can't." Your mind doesn't want you to be in shape.

That would require stress and pain. In reality, your mind will create any thought in your head to stop you from putting your body through the stress required to make the gains you desire. This makes consistent and disciplined training so difficult. In order to accomplish your goals, you have to learn to tame your mind. As you train, you soon realize there is a certain level of pain and suffering that must be endured to make gains. Well, that pain and discomfort is your body leaving its comfort zone. You must push through it. The bottom line is your mind will constantly try to keep you from pushing your body to and past that limit of comfort. You must overcome the overwhelming urge to quit. By doing so, you will then learn the secret of mind/body relationship.

These are the three aspects to becoming a "MACHINE." They are simple, yet not easily attained. This book provides you with one of the three elements. The other two elements rely strictly on your level of discipline.

So take this book, adopt a health diet geared towards what ever your goals are, and focus. Learn to push past the pain and train like a "MACHINE."

ABOUT THE AUTHOR

The author of this book is a long-time advocate of the fitness world. Spending most of his youth involved in competitive sports like wrestling, and track and field, he developed a strong passion for elite fitness early on. Throughout his life, he has continued his involvement in competitive sports, and he has also delved into the combative sport of mixed martial arts.

Though his passion for elite physical fitness is rooted mainly in sports, he also strives to achieve that synergetic pinnacle of endurance and strength for his personal goals as well as for his career. Bobby L. Clark is currently a Staff Noncommissioned Officer in the United States Marine Corps. As a Marine, his occupation is Firefighter. With such an extremely demanding profession, his physical and mental health are keys to his success.